C000175133

THE RESILIENCE TOOLKIT

*Powerful ways
to thrive in
blue-light services*

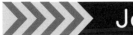 Jonathan Rees

Foreword by Chief Superintendent Ian Wylie

The Resilience Toolkit
Powerful ways to thrive in blue-light services
ISBN 978-1-912300-19-8
eISBN 978-1-912300-20-4

Published in 2019 by SRA Books

The right of Jonathan Rees to be identified as the author of
this work has been asserted by him in accordance with the
Copyright, Designs and Patents Act 1988.

Printed in the UK.

To all who are tired and worn out.

Contents

Foreword

Anyone embarking on a senior leadership role should expect it to be hard work and demanding. Senior leadership is a testing environment: managing multiple and complex issues; delivering an increasing portfolio of responsibilities; managing growing expectations of the public and customers; overseeing the relentless requirement for savings; responding to unpredictable and dynamic challenges and all the while maintaining the necessary forward momentum to meet your own performance objectives.

Sound familiar? Welcome to senior leadership and specifically senior leadership in the public sector. Since austerity began in 2011 public sector organisations have been shrinking year on year whilst at the same time demand for services has been growing relentlessly. You only need to think about the National Health Service winter crisis to understand that. The impact on senior leadership in this environment has been felt disproportionately, with the numbers of senior staff reduced significantly to help achieve those savings. Often the reduction in the number of senior leaders has been arbitrary based not on a sound evidence base of what senior leaders can reasonably be expected to deliver but instead based on 'finger in the air' planning where ever larger commands and portfolios become the norm with leaders 'just expected to deliver'.

Within UK policing and the realm of my own experience, this description is all too familiar to both me and my fellow senior operational leaders in the superintending ranks. Chief superintendents and superintendents are the backbone of senior police leadership and it is this cadre who lead the delivery of policing services across all corners of the UK. Their numbers have reduced by over 20 per cent since austerity began in 2011, the largest reduction of any rank in policing. Over the same period, and perhaps not surprisingly, their command responsibilities have grown exponentially placing significant demands on their own resilience. Regular surveys have illustrated worrying trends not only in terms of the requirement to increasingly work longer hours just to stand still but also increasing levels of poor physical and mental health.

Surviving and thriving in this 'pressure-cooker' environment is no small undertaking and following the last superintendents resilience survey in 2016, I commissioned Jonathan to develop a workshop programme for senior police leaders to help them do just that. To date over 500 superintendents and chief superintendents across the UK have benefited from these workshops which, equips them with the skills to deliver effectively in complex and extensive command environments. The feedback has been outstanding with colleagues now better equipped to deliver on a sustained basis under high pressure. This book represents the next stage of Jonathan's work and provides any senior leader in the public sector with an opportunity to learn and refresh the practical skills that will help them in these challenging roles. Whether you are a senior leader in policing, the NHS or elsewhere in the public sector I would recommend that you read this book and adopt its principles. I promise that it will help you to survive and thrive in the pressure cooker.

Best wishes,

Ian Wylie

Chief Superintendent
Vice-President, Police Superintendents' Association

Joff's story

Joff had always wanted to be a police officer, and now, lying in a hospital bed, he wondered if his dream was finally over. Chasing a car thief on foot, he'd followed him through a hedge only to plunge over a 15-foot drop. Concussed and with an arm and a leg in plaster as well as several titanium plates, he wasn't going to be going through an airport without raising attention ever again. Nor, and perhaps more sadly, he mused, was he going to be chasing a ball in the mud on Saturday afternoons with his friends.

Colleagues were kind enough to visit while he recovered, including his boss, bearing an unlikely looking gift. 'We've all got to read this,' he added, putting a large binder on the bedside locker.

With time to ponder his situation, he realised that while he might not chase criminals down the street again, he could still make a difference to people feeling safe. There had to be another role that he could fill. To his surprise, after a few days of utter boredom, Joff turned to the manual, and found it more interesting than he'd first imagined. The content just seemed to click for him, making sense as well as sparking ideas.

On returning to work, something came up relating to the binder's contents. 'You can't do that,' he told a colleague, 'the legislation won't allow it.'
'What legislation?'
'You know, the stuff in that binder.'
'Oh, yeah? Never read it myself.'

And with that, Joff realised that his new knowledge could plug a gap that others weren't able to fill.

Within a year, he was involved with making changes to the legislation, and he became quite influential. The challenge was, as the expert, everyone had to ask for his help, and it became more and more frustrating to him that no one was really paying attention. He saw his role as being as much to do with educating others about it as how to comply, and in time, some folk started working around him in order – as they saw it at least – to 'get the job done'.

With his favourite sporting outlet no longer available, stress and frustration built at work. So, he took all the coaching certificates possible for his sport, and started making a significant impact to his club's performance. But at work, relationships with some colleagues were still difficult.

Through an extended resilience coaching session, Joff explored how he could change his perception of his role, the purpose, and what others were trying to do. As a result, he shifted from an educational stance to an enabling one, drew clearer boundaries between his responsibilities and those of others, as well as between work and non-work. Consequently he's thriving again at work, and enjoying it more too.

Colleagues routinely comment on his demeanour and ask him what he's done. He just smiles.

Many organisations in commercial and public sectors, including police forces of the UK and Ireland, and indeed the UK Government, have identified an epidemic of wellbeing problems in the workplace (Stevenson/Farmer review, 2017).

Whether as a result of excessive workloads due to financial pressures or funding reductions, increased volumes of new types of work (such as cybercrime), or greater expectations brought about as a result of expected improvements in performance resulting from modern technology, the workplace has become a more stressful and challenging place to be. We need to know how to thrive in this pressure-cooker environment.

When I was working in the information technology (IT) industry from the late 1980s until the early 2000s, excessive working hours were the norm. Service providers and software development organisations were constantly trying to make a profit while being forced to sign fixed-price contracts against ill-defined requirements. Ultimately, it was the *people* who made it happen, as we all pulled together as a team.

At that point in my career, I used to leave home at 5.30 am every Monday and drive 230 miles to an office in Hull. We would work around 12 hours each day, and drive back home every Friday night – and this continued for almost 9 months. The work was challenging at times and everyone worked 50-plus hours a week, but I don't remember anyone ever being 'off sick', apart from the odd severe hangover! Something must have changed to create our current work problems.

I do not believe that wellbeing is the issue at hand today. That is not to say that there are no problems with people's wellbeing, nor that wellbeing programmes do not work; rather, that the *way* we are addressing these problems seems be focused on curing the symptoms rather than the cause. In the words of the learning and development director of one UK constabulary: 'We need to be working upstream of the problem.'

Life is unpredictable, and anything can go wrong for anyone at any time. Surely it would be better to enable people and organisations to handle the 'slings and arrows of outrageous fortune' and be ready for the unexpected, instead of just expecting them to routinely pick up the pieces?

The real problem is around *resilience*. We are not as resilient as we need to be.

Resilience is not some genetically inherited or mystical gift that some have while others do not. It is a multifaceted, dynamic and embedded part of being human, as much as it is a part of all living things. We are built to adapt. Some of us have adapted more than others, and in different ways.

People who are more resilient are able to handle the daily stresses of life calmly and more effectively. We all know people who find an inner strength when faced with a chaotic situation and, despite what is going on around them, have an ability to see the bigger picture, identify the critical actions necessary and just get things done.

However, this does not mean that they walk away from it unchanged. Often they find themselves completely drained and needing time to recuperate and process what happened. While we might think that experiencing challenging situations such as multi-vehicle road traffic collisions might have only negative impacts on those emergency service personnel involved, studies have shown that these experiences actually can build resilience – at least for some of us.

The impact of not being resilient is costly to individuals, organisations, families and society as a whole. High levels of resilience positively impact all of these contexts. In organisations where there is high complexity, risk and/or high rate of change, high resilience levels can have a positive effect.

The good news is that resilience can be developed. Enabling people to build (or rebuild) their resilience is more likely to have a significant impact on their wellbeing than head massages at their desk or away-days doing blind 4x4 driving – as enjoyable as these might be.

Given that this is such an important topic, you would expect there to be a consistent definition, but sadly there is not. With its roots in materials science, the earliest definitions of resilience are built around the ability to withstand physical loads. It also has been defined as an outcome, coping strategy and trait – which could include 'grit' and mindset, as the work and writing of Angela Duckworth and Carol Dweck attest.

One of the reasons for this lack of consistency is that resilience characteristics vary according to context – so there is research into the resilience of nurses, young children, adolescents, university students, yet a very limited amount on resilience in police officers, for example.

This variation means that there are equally numerous methods for measuring resilience. The most recent piece of research in this area comes from Dr Larry Mallak at the Western Michigan University, and includes this definition:

> In physical systems, resilience refers to a material's ability to store and return elastic energy. Similarly, in the workplace, we seek the ability for an employee to absorb energy from a stressful situation and to return to their original (or improved) condition once the stressor is removed. (Mallak and Yildiz, 2016)

As a keen runner, I was once extremely resilient biomechanically. Ten-mile training runs and regular long distances built up my physical resilience to be able to withstand the work required to complete a marathon in under 3 hours. Being physically fit and resilient led me to be more emotionally and mentally resilient: when I was running regularly, issues at work seemed more like bumps and potholes in the road than major issues and challenges.

It was quite a different story for a while though. I was injured with severe Achilles tendinitis, identified as being the result of an often-sedentary job, resulting in my gluteus maximus and minimus muscles becoming weakened. The effect was that while I could run at a 7-minute mile pace or better, I was unable to sustain the biomechanical control necessary for more than 2 miles – at which point my Achilles took all the strain and screamed in pain. There wasn't enough resilience in my physical body.

How did I know the cause? I consulted an expert in biomechanics – a physiotherapist, in other words – who assessed and diagnosed my condition and gave me a daily exercise regime to address the weakness. And because like many runners,

I feel out-of-sorts when missing my running, I worked hard at those drills to get back into my trainers as soon as I could.

Some days it was better, while some days it was worse again – but there was a definite upward trend, however slow. 'You know what this is going to be like,' my physio said at the last appointment. 'It'll be a mental and physical rollercoaster, but it will definitely improve.'

It seems a lot simpler to be thinking about resilience in physical terms than the modern working environment, yet there are useful patterns on which to draw.

One of the main challenges with resilience is that it is relative. Describing someone as resilient requires that we make a comparison – either against a previous time in their life, or against someone else. Both can be equally unhelpful. If it is relative, it is also contextual. My being less resilient physically has made me definitely less resilient emotionally, but it has not affected my resilience in other areas, such as being able to stand up in front of large groups of people and deliver keynote addresses.

Working with wood as I occasionally do, the evidence for adaptation to stress in trees is clear from the growth rings in the timbers I use – both their spacing and thickness. Dry seasons result in thinner rings, while the prevailing wind direction (and even gravity) can influence their spacing (Figure 1). In a similar way, our own nerve fibres show the impact of learning and adaptation, in the way that the myelin sheath wraps around the axon and increases the speed at which nerve signals can travel (Figure 2).

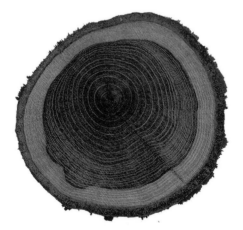

Figure 1: Cross-section of laburnum branch showing growth rings

One psychological definition of resilience is 'the role of mental processes and behaviour in promoting personal assets and protecting an individual from the potential negative effect of stressors' (Fletcher and Sarkar, 2013). While this is helpful in terms of including both mental and behavioural aspects, it does not define the actual characteristic itself.

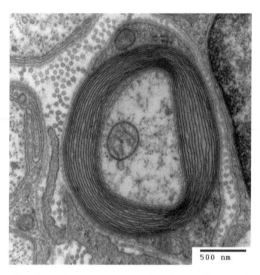

Figure 2: Cross-section through a neutron showing the myelin sheath

Therefore, for the purposes of this book, I am going to take this definition from Warner and April in 'Building personal resilience at work' (2012), which describes resilience as:

> that developed characteristic for dealing with negative and positive changes in life, accessible to all people on a daily basis, which distinguishes survivors/adaptors (employing successful, regular adaptation, and drawing from internal and external sources of strength usually associated with the psychological concept of having a bi-local locus of control) from those who give in to life's struggles (often resulting in pathological and, normally negative, life-adjusting effects)...

While this is quite a challenging statement for those of us who find our resilience to be low, it incorporates the adaptive 'bounce-back' characteristic that people most commonly point to when asked what resilience is, while also including the ability to emerge stronger from times of trial.

My outcome for you

I strongly believe that this is too important a subject to continue to leave to chance, with a lot of the information residing in academia. Today's workplace is fast-paced, highly complex and even life-threatening at times. As a society, we are placing ever-increasing burdens on our security and emergency services, while expecting them just to absorb them. You only have to watch a TV documentary filmed from the perspective of paramedics or police officers to get a glimpse into how much resilience is required.

This is not a new idea. It is one that we have forgotten as we have elevated the need for personal success – whether financial or material – above that of learning for the future and how to live together well. However, we cannot live together well until we do something about behaviour that is driven from an avoidance of failure or loss-of-face that features in nearly every area of business and politics, leading to guilt, shame and, it seems, lower interpersonal connections, in turn leading to diminishing hopefulness.

We live in challenging times. It has always been that way. Rather than railing against it, is it not time to accept where we find ourselves, and move forward? It is a bit like trekking to base camp on Everest, where the altitude and reduced air pressure means that water boils at a lower temperature and so your cup of tea does not brew the same as at home. It doesn't taste how we want it, but it is still hot, wet and gives you the same physical benefits – probably!

I am guessing, as best any author can, that you are interested in this subject from a personal or leadership perspective. Perhaps you are a superintendent within an emergency service, or a senior manager in a commercial organisation. Or maybe the title piqued your curiosity as to how you might build greater resilience. My hope is that you will find something useful and thought-provoking within these pages.

With such variation in context and definition, my aim is to combine multiple strands of thinking, research and experience: whether that is due to advances in neuroscience and the massive increase in our understanding of the brain; or whether it is reflecting on the impact of technology, social media and on-demand entertainment.

I have tried to make this book accessible for multiple styles of reading – there is no one-size-fits-all or silver-bullet answer to this challenge. So this book can be read front to back, or you can dip in and out, selecting tools that you like the look of.

While this is a physical or electronic book, it cannot replace a multi-week training programme – and it is not intended to do so. Instead, the aim is to explore the facets of this complex human characteristic, in the hope that you will be able to choose the factors that are most personally relevant, and start exploring how you might begin to change. You would do well to do that in conjunction with one-to-one coaching support – preferably from someone who does not have a detailed understanding of your work context, as they will ask wider questions to broaden your thinking. (We will come back to coaching later.)

I believe that we all have the right to enjoy rather than just endure work. That it *is possible* to thrive in the pressure cooker of modern work life. I hope that you'll enjoy joining me as we explore these various 'ingredients'.

A note before we continue: many of the principles here are illustrated through stories. These are often a fusion of real events that I have experienced or heard about. All names given are fictitious, and any resemblance to a real person is unintended.

Health warnings

This is not a psychological textbook, neither does it aim to provide advice on dealing with issues such as post-traumatic stress disorder (PTSD) or other mental health conditions. Please consult a medical practitioner rather than relying on this book, if this applies to you.

Also please consult your doctor first before starting any exercise programme suggested or listed in this book, especially if you have any pre-existing conditions.

Part 1: An integrated model

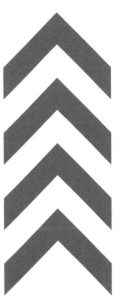

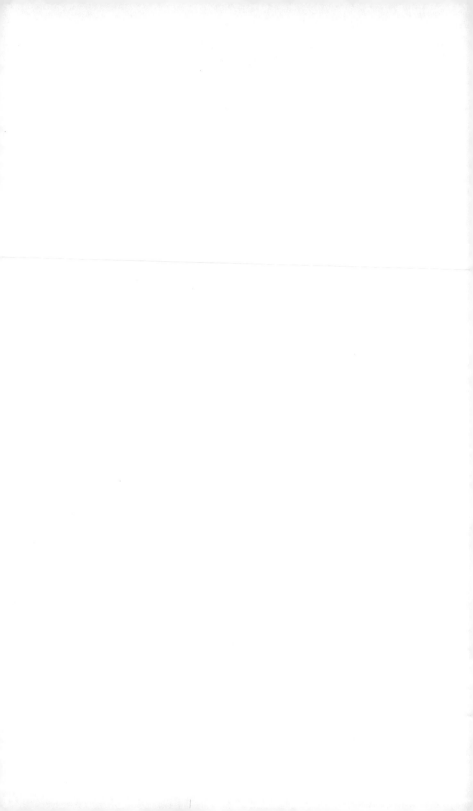

1. Background

While exploring resilience, I searched for academic papers and books across multiple genres such as biology, psychology and business. As I did so, it became clear that there are many different viewpoints on what resilience is, and how we can build it as we seek to thrive. It quickly became clear that instead of having multiple definitions, we need a model that draws these strands together.

People often ask: 'Isn't resilience really just about *coping* better?' Coping is definitely one element of resilience, but it is not the whole picture. One model (proposed by Weiten and Lloyd, 2008) describes coping in terms of three viewpoints:

- Adaptive focus
- Problem focus
- Emotion focus

These can be considered as three separate strategies.

- Adaptive strategies – changing how we *think* and *feel* about a challenging situation by using a technique to gain a different viewpoint.
- Constructive strategies – finding ways to *change* a situation by reducing the stressful impact that it has on us, or by eliminating it altogether. This includes looking for previously unseen benefits, by considering what we might *learn* from the situation.
- Proactive strategies – techniques to *prepare* ourselves for challenges in advance.

The first two of these strategies are about reacting to challenging situations when we find ourselves within them, while the third is about preparing for them, whether anticipated or unexpected.

There are some things that we can do that will contribute to our ability to be resilient during a challenging event, while there are also those that we can do to build our resilient capacity in advance. I will refer to these as *reactive resilience* and *proactive resilience*. For the sake of clarity, I do not differentiate between the tools and techniques that contribute to either (or both) within the integrated model.

As we have established, resilience is more than just coping. It also includes having access to (and therefore building) tools and techniques to prepare for, and deal with, both negative and positive life changes. There is a clear difference between those things that lie outside us that affect our resilience and those that lie within us, and so we can group these into three factors, as shown in Figure 3:

- Cognitive (thinking) – the pupil
- Behavioural – the iris
- Relational – the eye itself

The resilience model

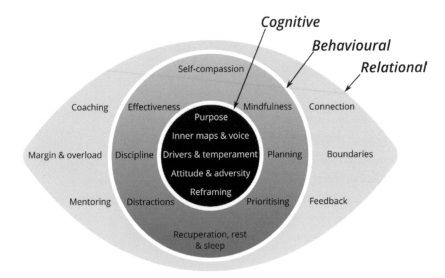

Figure 3: An integrated model of resilience

This model maps well with the self-efficacy model as proposed by Albert Bandura in 1986. Although now more than 40 years old, this is all about believing that we have the ability to organise ourselves and act appropriately to manage a situation, and has three dimensions:

- Internal personal factors
- Behaviour
- External environment

I have chosen to place Bandura's 'affective' and 'biological' events within the behavioural factors to distinguish more strongly that the innermost trait-like factors are the starting point for all resilience building. Therefore, this book is structured into cognitive, behavioural and relational factors.

Before we get into the details of each factor, it is important to examine what other work has been done in the area of training for resilience. A systematic review of 14 different workplace resilience training programmes carried out in 2015 (by Robertson, Cooper, et al.) showed that most programmes took a cognitive-behavioural approach, for example: workshops on relaxation techniques, mental rehearsal, optimism, emotional intelligence, mindfulness and stress reduction.

The review looked at four key resilient contexts:

- Mental health and subjective wellbeing
- Psychosocial outcomes
- Physical/biological outcomes
- Performance outcomes

While it was clear that resilience training does work, and has other benefits such as improving performance, no firm conclusions could be drawn on which was the most effective content and format, and that the 'empirical evidence was tentative except for a large effect for mental health and subjective well-being' (Robertson, Cooper, et al., 2015).

Some of the studies reviewed even showed that having initially higher levels of resilience may reduce the impact of additional resilience training – almost as if having the belief that we do not need to improve our resilience makes us more resistant to doing so! The method used for the training also affects the outcomes achieved: for example, online resilience training did not have any impact at all.

Linking to the three-factor structure used here, it is interesting to note that providing one-to-one support such as coaching and/or mentoring – often excluded from corporate training programmes due to cost constraints – is seen as being important. These two topics are included as part of the relational factors.

2. A resilience factor

'If you know the enemy and know yourself, you need not fear the result of a hundred battles. If you know yourself but not the enemy, for every victory gained you will also suffer a defeat. If you know neither the enemy nor yourself, you will succumb in every battle.'

Sun Tzu

Over the last 30 years, many resilience instruments have been designed, researched and tested. Most are aimed at very specific contexts (e.g. PTSD to nursing) or life stages (e.g. child to university student). Only one, which also happens to be the most recent, has been created and refined specifically for the workplace: the Workplace Resilience Instrument (WRI) by Dr Larry Mallak (2018). Dr Mallak has kindly given permission for the WRI to be included in this book (see the Resources section).

The WRI measures four dimensions of workplace resilience:

1. Active problem-solving – having a predisposition to action rather than focusing on the source of a difficult situation.
2. Team efficacy – having an understanding of how other people experience the world, how they work in teams and on shared goals.
3. Confident sense-making – making sense of a situation in a calm, focused and confident manner, especially one that is chaotic.
4. Bricolage – having the ability to use available tools, methods and materials to solve a problem in a creative way.

These are essentially what the resilience literature refers to as 'protective' factors – i.e. those that can enable a person to increase their resilience, as opposed to their vulnerability. Usefully, Mallak and Yildiz (2016) compared the results of their instrument against an established job stress questionnaire (the Brief Job Stress Questionnaire – BJSQ), which considers three factors:

- Job control – how much control someone has over the task they are given
- Support – how much help or assistance they get to do it
- Job demand – the volume of work required

One naturally would expect that each of these stress factors would be reduced when we have higher resilience. However, it turns out that people having higher levels of resilience actually experience higher 'job demand' stress, which suggests that someone with higher resilience experiences these stresses – due to overload, work–life balance and conflict challenges – differently to someone with lower resilience.

When people have higher resilience, they obviously have less sickness absence. People who are more resilient also act more effectively in the event of a crisis, make better quality decisions and, overall, have higher satisfaction from their work – so they thrive.

Knowing the contexts within which we are least resilient enables us to make effective improvements to those areas. It is important to be aware of the areas within which we are *most* resilient as – following the principles of Appreciative Inquiry – it may be far easier to make improvements by building on what already works well. As David Cooperrider, co-founder of the theory of Appreciative Inquiry, states: 'The appreciative mode awakens the desire to create and discover new social possibilities that can enrich our existence and give it meaning' (2013).

Next step

1. Find out your resilience factor using the Workplace Resilience Instrument now (see the Resources section).

3. Compounding

How to use this book

> 'Little actions repeated relentlessly result in big change. Don't underestimate the importance of "small" multiplied by "often".'
>
> David Hieatt

It is entirely up to you how you will use this book. There are many factors covered here that can contribute to building a resilient life and thriving, and it would be impossible for you to do something in-depth about each of them.

Instead, we can learn from sport and think about it like compound interest. Dave Brailsford was the manager of the UK cycling team that swept the board with gold medals at the 2016 Olympics. He focused the team on marginal gains – tiny changes that, individually, did not amount to much until compounded together, when they became more significant. For example, the team took their own pillows to hotels to ensure that they slept better.

As you read this book, just notice what particularly resonates with you, as well as what does not. Make notes on the areas that, while initially appearing to be just a small change to your routine or thinking patterns, could have a significant effect on your resilience when consistently repeated over time.

When you reach the end of the book, transcribe the top five or six things that you are going to start with onto a sticky note or index card. The action of writing will embed it in your mind better than just highlighting it, and you will most likely find that, three months from now, things have changed for the better. Then you can try out some other ideas, and so on.

Let's get started.

Next step

1. Most chapters will end with a thought or two for you to get on with and apply what has been described. Some have accompanying worksheets, videos or even online training modules. If you want to access them, go to the-resilience-toolkit.com and register your copy of this book.

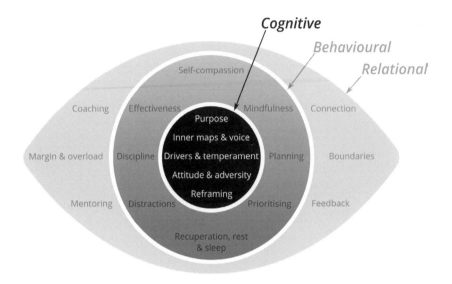

Part 2: Cognitive factors

4. Purpose

'Purpose is a powerful business tool. Both for the business you want to grow and the change you want to make. Purpose allows you to know why it matters, why your time on this crazy thing isn't wasted. Which reduces stress.'

The Stress Report

Gandhi and the sugar

A woman once went to Mahatma Gandhi and asked him to tell her overweight son to stop eating sugar. 'Madam,' he replied, 'come back in three weeks' time.'

Surprised at this request, she nevertheless returned with her son three weeks later and repeated her question. Gandhi looked at the boy and said: 'Boy. Stop eating sugar.'

When the boy had left the room, the mother turned to Gandhi and asked why he had not said this three weeks before. 'Madam, three weeks ago I myself was eating sugar.'

Be the change

If we want to see a change in our world, we have to start with ourselves. To get our own house in order. The inner show of our life runs the outer show, and hence the point of greatest leverage. But where should we start when considering that inner show?

In most organisations, when we are not getting the results we need, we go through a process of identifying gaps, using those to identify training needs, provide appropriate training and then expect the gaps to close. Yet often this approach does not seem to work as well as we think it should. There is always *some* improvement, of course, and we usually justify the remaining gap as being due to the quality of training, the environment or other factors beyond our control. However, very rarely do we put it down to the participant. Either way, this is unsatisfactory. What if there were a way to get a better result, maybe at lower cost of money and time?

We can turn this situation on its head and look at performance through a different lens. Instead of focusing on ability, we can focus on thinking.

Consider this model: the Performance Pyramid, based on Robert Dilts' 'logical-levels' model, which I first encountered while training in Neuro Linguistic Programming (NLP) (Figure 4).

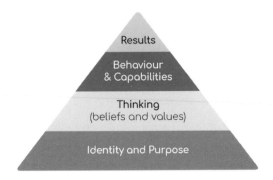

Figure 4: The Performance Pyramid

This model shows that by having greater clarity on our purpose and our identity within a given context, our thinking changes. When that happens, our behaviour and capabilities change, and so do our results.

What is important about this is the leverage from bottom to top: with only a small change in our thinking we can have a greater impact on the behaviour and results we achieve. So, greater clarity on our purpose and identity has greater impact than capability development alone.

Identity shifting created a runner

When I talk about running marathons, a lot of people make comments to the effect that they hate running, they hated it at school, find it boring and so on. Indeed, I don't recall enjoying the prospect of the annual school cross-country race either. I only took up running after my colleague Judy loaned me a book (Jim Fixx's *Complete Book of Running*). Having nothing better to do that evening, I sat down to read and finished it at around 1.30 am.

I decided that if running would give me only a fraction of the benefits that Fixx described, I had to try it. So, off I went in tatty gym kit. I turned left at the end of the road, left and left again, until I got home a couple of miles later. When I finished, I remembered sitting on the grass beside the athletics track at school with a sense of 'I must do this', accompanied by the thought 'I'll save up for some of those spiked shoes'.

Taking up running changed my life forever. Within a month I signed up for a half-marathon, and ran 10 of them within the next year. I got the spiked shoes, and ran proper cross-country, in mud, rain, hail and ice falling from trees at the start line of one race. I loved it – I still do. For me, there is nothing better than running in whatever weather, whether in the city or the country. I am at one with myself, and the created world around me.

How did this happen? How did I, a confirmed non-runner, become so committed to this sport? Reading that book shifted my purpose and identity that day. I didn't go to the gym to build my strength or take up a training programme. I just got out and did it. Shifting your purpose, identity, and beliefs can massively shift the results you get.

When thinking about our resilience, this has one main implication: clarity of purpose is critical, as it drives everything else.

What is your 'why'?

In the words of organisational consultant Simon Sinek (2009), 'A failure to communicate why creates nothing but stress or doubt... Absent a why, a decision is harder to make.' By 'why' here, Sinek means 'purpose', 'higher cause', 'belief' or 'value'. Notice how these all overlap with the bottom half of the Performance Pyramid.

Having a clear 'why' enables us to make better decisions, aligned decisions. It also enables us to take a step back when things change, as they inevitably do.

Beginning with the end in mind is one of my watchwords from Stephen Covey's great *The 7 Habits of Highly Effective People* (2004). It too is about having a clear purpose.

I had long expected purpose to be key to being more resilient because of the Performance Pyramid. I wasn't surprised, therefore, to find some research done in 2009 by Jenny Campbell, in *Resilience in Personal and Organisational Life*. Campbell interviewed 25 c-suite managers and uncovered that one of the key factors enabling their resilience was having a clear, outward-focused purpose for their life. This enabled them to transcend the frequent oscillations that the rest of us perform between coping and bouncing back.

Having a strong sense of purpose enables 'breakthrough resilience' – a 'state of energised, resourceful adaptability, where day-to-day challenges are seen relative to achievement of a strongly personal future state and thus have less significance' (Campbell, 2009). What is more, having pushed through to this state, the managers found that it was such a compelling place to be that they worked hard to remain there.

Keeping your eye on the destination

One of my friends, Mark, loves to sail.

'The thing about sailing is, apart from the sheer exhilaration of being propelled across the sea or a lake by only the power of nature, that you have to keep your eye on where you want to end up, and make constant adjustments to the sails to make sure you get there. If the wind is coming straight at you from your destination, then you have to tack across it from time to time.

That might look like a zig-zag path to someone watching from the shore, but to you it's just keeping your eye on the goal, and adjusting and tweaking things until you get there – and when you do, there's usually a nice, cool beer to relax with!'

None of this is easy, of course. Otherwise you would not be reading this book, and I would not be writing it – we would just be enjoying ourselves somewhere. I hope that you can see its importance clearly now. When we have a significant personal purpose (SPP) – one that goes far beyond ourselves – we are able to bring a strong focus to bear on it, and other things fall away.

Having an SPP is more of a protective factor than a reactive one. Knowing this should encourage us to spend the time to get really clear on it. Then we will be able to pause in challenging situations and choose to see them as enablers to help us achieve, or recognise them as less significant and just bumps in the road.

Next steps

1. What is your SPP? Use your values, beliefs and higher cause to identify it.

2. Go to the-resilience-toolkit.com to register your copy of this book and get a guided exercise to identify your purpose at work.

3. Take the largest piece of paper you can find. In silence, draw a picture, without words, that represents how you want life to be for you in six months' time.

5. Inner maps

'Resilience is built on the simple realisation that our emotions and behaviours are triggered not by events themselves, but how we interpret those events.'

(Reivich and Shatté, 2003)

The way we think about what is happening, what has happened, and what may happen to us has a much greater influence on our resilience than we believe. So it is useful to explore those thinking patterns, and their impact on our resilience.

Thinking out loud in silence

Depending on our personality, experiences and upbringing, there are a number of different factors that influence how we experience the real world through our thinking. One of the most obvious is whether we internalise or externalise that process. Some of us prefer considering aspects of a situation alone, writing down our thoughts; while others (myself included) prefer stream-of-consciousness discussions to explore different facets, and may not make any written notes at all.

Depending on which you prefer, you may find people who take the opposite approach to be immensely frustrating, or even alarming. They seem to meander through the conversation, going down blind alleys only to retrace their mental perambulations seconds, minutes or even hours later.

If you are someone who likes this style of 'think-talking', you can feel guilty that it takes a while to come into land on any decision. You find the silent cogitation of the self-talkers frustrating, as it seems to make no progress. While you are thinking, 'Surely two heads are better than one?', they are thinking, 'When can we stop talking so I can go away and think?' Both are equally valid, of course – they are just different.

A shift in thinking

Peter, one of my team, was due to take an extended holiday. He was working out a plan to share his responsibilities to others during his time away, including me.

> Struggling to get that done alongside the demands of the rest of his day job, we chatted it through over a cup of coffee. I asked a few questions as we explored things from a number of different angles, when he suddenly looked up.
>
> 'I'm so sorry, I really should have thought this all through before. I've just not had the time – and I know that I'm meant to come to everything with solutions instead of answers, so this is probably very frustrating to just be talking and darting all over the place. You must think I'm mad.'
>
> His inner map – created by upbringing and past experience – was that people who talk things through are just indecisive. 'It's fine,' I replied, 'we're all uniquely made, with our own best ways of thinking.'

Representing the world

> 'The map is not the territory.'
>
> (Korzybski, 1995)

However we approach thinking, we are subject to how our senses gather data about the world, and how our brains represent it to us. Our senses provide a constant stream of information to our brains, at a rate estimated to exceed 2Mb/sec. While that is not enough to stream an episode of our favourite TV series, it is utterly overwhelming to our thinking engine, which can process only an estimated 134b/sec. So our brain applies a process of filtering. It filters out information that seems unnecessary, and we extrapolate meaning using information that we have stored from earlier experiences – which opens up the risk of misrepresentation later on, as we know only too well.

All our internal representations depend on, and consist of, these five core components:

- Pictures – visual
- Sounds – auditory
- Feelings, both inner and outer – kinaesthetic
- Smell – olfactory
- Taste – gustatory

We each have a preference for how we experience the world through one of these components. Most of us prefer to use visual methods. Olfactory and gustatory preferences are rare in Western culture.

With a preference for one of these, we will tend to not notice the other elements of a situation. No doubt you will have experienced this when you have been to the cinema with a group of friends.

> 'I loved that film. A rich storyline, and very believable characterisations,' says one.
>
> 'I was bored, I didn't make a connection with any of the characters,' says another.
>
> 'I agree – not a good film, often inappropriate music which confused me,' adds a third.

Each is correct, and just demonstrating their particular communication preference.

Uncomfortable *Spectre*

About a week after the James Bond film *Spectre* opened, we took a family trip to the cinema. While I was getting drinks and snacks, the rest of the family found that the only available space was in the front row. I ended up with a seat by the wall.

As a result of having to move my head to reduce the parallax error, and leaning backwards slightly due to the proximity of the screen, my only recollection after the opening chase is one of discomfort.

Awareness of these traits allows you to increase your flexibility by purposefully noticing them. When we do this, we often have a flash of inspiration that leads to rapid resolution of a situation and awareness of our feelings.

In the same way that we differ in how we perform thinking, we also build our own unique filters, some of which are listed below.

Filter
Attached/Detached
Proactive/Reactive
Towards/Away

Filter
Internal/External
Similarity/Difference
Big picture/Small picture

While this seems rather complicated, the point is to illuminate the fact that each can influence how we respond to events, and having an increased awareness of them provides us with an opportunity to choose the most useful response when faced with challenging situations.

We all have a bias to interpret what we experience as justifying or supporting existing beliefs. This can lead us to draw false conclusions about whether or not we can get through a difficult situation. If we conclude that we cannot, then we will not even try to bring energy to bear on the problem, and may allow ourselves to be overcome. As before, this is completely personal and may be context-specific. The stories that we tell ourselves can be extremely powerful, affecting not only ourselves but also our relationships with others.

Let's explore these filters by starting with how we perceive ourselves in our world – from either a detached perspective or an attached one.

Attached or detached?
When we take a detached perspective, we see ourselves within our world from the viewpoint of a third party. We can see and hear everything around us, behind and above us, but we have no reliable experience of feelings, and are unable to sense inner thoughts.

An attached perspective views the world solely as we can sense it, and includes a full range of sensory information – but like a blind person examining an elephant, we have limitations.

Imagine riding a bicycle. With a detached view, we can see the back wheel in its entirety. Taking an attached view, we cannot – at least not without dropping our head down to look backwards, usually resulting in spilt blood, a damaged machine and dented pride.

When we recognise that we tend to associate *into* experiences, it is helpful to imagine taking a step back and seeing more of the situation. If our preference is to dissociate *from* a situation, associating *into* it can help us to be more empathic, and also provides us with useful information.

Proactive or reactive?

> 'Reactive people do not believe that they control their world. Chances are that they will be waiting for someone else to solve problems for them.'
>
> Shelle Rose Charvet

Taking an active approach to problem-solving is a key attribute that provides resilience. While a proactive person believes they have some control over events, a reactive person does not.

With a preference towards a proactive stance, we respond to a situation early and get on with it without waiting for others to act. However, this can sometimes cause us to act too quickly and without sufficient thought. While this is better than freezing, there is a balance to be struck – a resilient leader will want to take the most appropriate action without analysis paralysis.

On the other hand, strong reactive tendencies may cause us to hesitate and to wait for others to take action, freezing, or waiting to see what is going to happen next and delaying action. This may appear as not making a decision, but failing to act is a decision in itself.

BRAN

Attending National Childbirth Trust (NCT) classes with my wife before the birth of our first child, we were taught an acronym to use when a quick decision is necessary during a birth – BRAN:

- What is the *Best* thing to do
- The *Recommended* thing to do
- The *Alternatives*
- The likely impact of doing *Nothing*

Towards or away?

This thinking pattern is about our direction of focus – either towards a goal, or away from a problem.

Having a strong 'away-from' motivation may cause us to focus on only how to stop a difficult situation occurring, instead of being more resilient and taking action to deal with it. Taken to its extreme, this could result in trying to avoid blame or shame, which can make us less resilient in the long term because of concerns over being discovered later. A strong 'away-from' motivation provides a positive desire to solve an urgent problem, but that can lead to difficulties in prioritisation of non-urgent activities.

A strong 'towards' motivation can also impact our resilience, because focusing only on the desired end-state may compromise our opportunities to learn. Hence a balance is required between these two extremes – a resilient person is goal-oriented while also having effective problem-solving skills.

Having high bricolage (the ability to use available tools, methods and materials to solve a problem in a creative way) means we are able to achieve this balance by using the tools and resources at our disposal, rather than feeling helpless, and we are therefore more resilient.

Internal or external?

This thinking pattern is about what we use as our point of reference. Those of us who are internally referenced have our own inner standards against which we compare ourselves, while an externally referenced person makes comparisons against provided standards. Of course, this can apply just as much to how resilient we believe we are, as it does to how we judge the quality of our work.

Internally referenced folk do not ignore the available information, they just make decisions based on their own internal standards. Conversely, externally referenced folk may require others not only to set standards, but also judge whether they are being met.

From external to internal referencing

Jeff was a software developer in one of my project teams. Technically brilliant, and highlighted as a talent for the future, his external referencing was so strong that he would check technical decisions with me before finally implementing them.

My approach was always to take a coaching stance.

'How would you judge this from a technical standpoint?'
'Does this break new technical ground for us?'
'What's the relative risk compared to a tried-and-tested – though lower performance – solution?'

> In time, Jeff started to ask himself these questions and trust his own
> intuition. He shifted towards being more internally referenced.

From a resilient stance, both extremes have downsides. Strong *external* referencing can result in freezing rather than taking an active decision. Strong *internal* referencing may see us acting only according to our own standards, and ignoring the feedback inherent in any challenging situation. We also lose a learning opportunity.

Seeking similarity or demanding difference?

We are all making constant comparisons. In every situation, some of us notice what matches our prior experiences and existing knowledge, while others are more aware of what is different or does not match. Both viewpoints are equally valid; however, myopia in either direction can be frustrating to someone with the opposite predisposition (Figure 5).

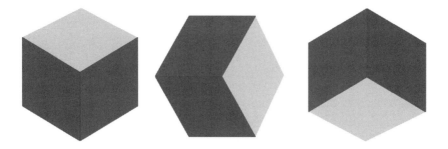

Figure 5: Three cubes

Do these three cubes look the same to you? You may see three cubes that are all the same – because of their size. Or all the same but different because they are rotated, or all different because they are all rotated, or all different and the same size. Unlike the other filtering we have already considered, this is less clear-cut, as when we sort for similarity or difference, there are nuances:

- All the same (pure sameness)
- Same with differences
- Different (pure difference)
- Different with similarities

Which of these we notice tells us something about our level of comfort and desire for change.

If we sort for 'pure sameness', we will tend to seek situations in which there is little change: for example, resisting the introduction of new technology. If we notice 'same with differences', then we are comfortable with and may seek gradual change – a late adopter of new technology.

Conversely, if we sort for 'pure difference', then change is our thing – we get bored more easily than most, and are often early adopters. If at first we are aware of difference then similarities, we will be looking for the uniqueness of the early adopter, but just off the cutting edge.

If we consider that part of resilience as the ability to respond usefully in times of change, then knowing where we sit on the spectrum of demanding difference or seeking similarity can forewarn us as to the depth of challenge that we are going to face. If we have a predisposition to either extreme, it may be important for us to find allies who can temper our extremes. Although the challenges for a 'sameness' person are obvious, those who notice difference may be tempted to adopt a novel solution when there is a perfectly suitable and proven one already to hand.

(In case you're wondering, the second cube is rotated 90° and flipped, the third is just rotated 180°.)

Big picture or little details?

This filter probably causes more misunderstandings than any we have considered so far. Some of us are wired to think and observe the general situation, while others catch the minutiae and finer detail of what is going on (closely aligned with the iNtuitive vs Sensing factors in the Myers Briggs Type Indicator (MBTI)).

He doesn't do detail...

Unusually, I arrived at the meeting 5 minutes early, and as I pushed the door open, heard 'But that's the problem, he just doesn't do detail, he...' cut off mid-flow when the speaker – James – saw me.

I considered myself able to 'do detail'. It was just that my role demanded that I take a more strategic standpoint: one which saw the forest rather than the individual trees.

Even as I am writing this, I notice my inner voice reminding me of when I *do* 'do detail' – making things in my workshop or repairing broken

---

equipment, for example. What are those activities, if they're not 'doing detail'? Is that not sufficient evidence?

Of course James was not commenting on my ability or otherwise to do detail across the whole of my life, just the context within which he saw me at work. I could have responded with: 'But the problem we have is that you constantly pull us down into the weeds...' Fortunately, that wasn't the day for having a barney with James.

Those of us with a natural pull towards the bigger picture and generalities of a situation are comfortable thinking in and handling big 'chunks' – strategic activities and the like. We can find small detail overwhelming, so we may brush over and ignore details that others would not miss. Our breadth of vision of a situation may lead us to share thoughts about it in a rather random way – fine for us, but sometimes irritating for others.

If we are drawn towards thinking and working with smaller chunks, we need lots of detail to be able to make sense of the whole picture. We want to break things down into discrete steps or defined processes, even if the whole situation is so large that we can only determine the single next step.

As always, there are strengths and weaknesses associated with this filtering pattern. Miscommunication is most likely when those of us who prefer general and strategic information find ourselves bored and overwhelmed with what we see as unnecessary details, and so summarise a situation from our viewpoint. Our detail-oriented colleagues may then add more and more detail to (as they see it) enable the strategist to 'get it', only leading to circular discussions and escalating tension.

In a challenging situation which demands resilience, both viewpoints have their benefits. Each needs to act as 'control rods' to one another, so that neither do we become stuck as a result of seeking more detail, but nor do we brush aside what may turn out to be important details for responding optimally.

Walking a mile in another man's shoes
Each of these filtering perspectives has clear benefits as well as disadvantages. It is important to know which ones we naturally use, and to learn how to switch between them to enrich our maps.

This is an essential skill when we are building rapport with others, especially those with whom we do not see eye-to-eye. Walking in the other person's shoes always gives us a different and valuable perspective – and in a challenging situation, having the flexibility to adjust, or knowing that we need to draw on someone else when we cannot, means that we cope rather than sink.

It can be useful to remember that all these facets are in play when we are considering how to interpret, react to and anticipate, future challenges. We can help one another to be more resilient by remembering that reality is more about how we interpret and respond to events, rather than the actual events themselves. By being more aware of each, and our personal predispositions, we can shift our perspective faster and thus be more action-focused, make faster decisions and, ultimately, be more resilient. Moreover, when we are not in the midst of such challenges, we can use our self-awareness to rehearse flexing to an alternative viewpoint, so that we are ready when the need does arise.

Next steps

1. Carefully consider each of the filters we have explored here, decide which is most like you and which you have the most difficulty adopting. Choose one to practise shifting to for a week at a time, and notice by journalling what is different as a result.
2. Think about a challenging situation, and decide which filters are going to be the most helpful, and which the least. Use your self-awareness from (1) to plan how you are going to flex – or who you could draw on to assist you.

6. Inner voice

'Internal verbalisations are the talk and chatter that constantly invade the human consciousness while internal visualisations are mental pictures that are produced in the human mind. Therapists believe both need taming.'

(Pulla, 2013)

Emotional intelligence

Increasing our awareness of the 'internal verbalisations' as Venkat Pulla describes them here – which I shall refer to as 'inner voice' – is at the heart of emotional intelligence (EQ).

People with strong EQ are good at five key things, according to Daniel Goleman:

- being aware of their emotions
- managing them – and sharing appropriately
- harnessing them productively
- having empathy for others
- handling relationships.

In challenging situations, when emotions run high, we need to be able to apply these skills and then return to an even keel when the event has passed. It is not about not feeling stuff, but about controlling the effect it has on us and expressing it appropriately without losing sight of the goal – and then taking action, regardless.

I have only ever met one person who believed that they did not have this constant 'inner chatter'. For some of us, it is perhaps something that we just need to tune into; perhaps it is also something to do with context.

We're going to die...

Martin is a keen cyclist (he only just missed selection for a place in the Tour de France). He told me how, throughout his racing career, he had thought that he was the only person in the peloton with constantly competing inner thoughts while racing. On one shoulder was the voice

---

> that said 'Wow, this is really fun, and so fast!', while on the other a
> different 'voice' was screaming 'Help, we're going to all die!'
>
> He only discovered it was true for all of them, when he happened to
> mention it to a good friend.

This inner voice shows the amazing ability of our observational powers.

> **Simultaneous strands**
>
> After playing and singing at a particularly uplifting church meeting
> recently, I was chatting with Adam the keyboard player. I remarked
> how I had noticed during one particular song a neat pattern that the
> drummer was playing, and that I had changed my strumming pattern
> to match.
>
> What we both found remarkable was that I was aware of this happen-
> ing through a narrative that was running in part of my brain at the
> same time as I was reading music, fingering chords and singing the
> right words, as well as listening to the other instruments.

This happens in many areas of our lives. Think about the last time you were giving a presentation. Most likely, your inner dialogue was saying things like: 'This
is good, they all seem to be paying attention', or 'Oh, look at the time, I need to
speed up', or even 'That woman in the back of the room looks familiar, where do
I know her from – is it…?'

Talk to any climbers you know, for example. They will tell you that during a climb,
their mind becomes wonderfully free and clear. One described it to me as: 'Pure
mindfulness, as I can only think about where the next hand or foothold is going to
be.' There are precious few moments in modern life when this happens, and we
need to seek them out if we are to hear this inner voice.

When the chatter is positive, we can take advantage of its energy and drive to
keep us moving forward and encourage ourselves and others. With the increase
in EQ that it gives us, we can observe the emotional state of other people and
reflect that back to them in appropriate ways. When the chatter turns negative or
judgemental, we can catch it, challenge it and turn it around.

Interpreting our inner voice

It is important to realise that what we interpret as an instruction from our inner voice is only an offer. We do not have to act on it, although we do have to manage it if we want to avoid ending up with inner warfare between the animal and human parts of our brain. One innate human ability is responsiveness – the ability to choose how we respond, or be response-able. Because the interconnections within our brain are driven by chemical exchange, there is a finite time (1/10th second) during which we can decide to pause and take a more balanced view.

Choosing to be mad

After a lengthy discussion with a very senior Hewlett-Packard IT manager about how to solve an impasse on a project, I got off the phone in a foul mood.

Storming over to the coffee machine, as I waited for the cup to fill, I noticed my inner (animal) voice chattering away grumpily. What was the most useful thing to do? Be mad, or let it go?

I decided to be mad for 10 minutes, then get back on with my work.

Recognising that the inner voice is always telling us stories helps us remember that we may not be correct in our conclusions. The brain makes up stories based on limited information, and fills in the gaps using information from our beliefs and values. We use these stories to drive our interactions with one another, and our relationships can suffer as a result.

Professor Brené Brown specialises in the area of vulnerability. In *Rising Strong*, she talks about two key steps to start changing this:

1. The reckoning – realising what is going on for us emotionally, and the possibility that the stories we are telling ourselves may not be completely accurate.
2. The rumble – boldly stepping into situations and talking about the stories we are telling ourselves.

This led me to the idea of practising 'ask and tell', which is about sharing the stories that we are telling ourselves with those involved, and allowing them to correct and reassure us when we are wide of the mark.

Increased awareness of our inner stories enables us to control and change them. It also enables us to become aware of patterns and the contexts within which they arise, so that we can be better prepared in the future. Moreover, paying attention to the language itself is useful. Often, we find that the inner dialogue is harsh and judgemental: just think about the last time you were doing something and it wasn't going very well, despite having done it before or trained for it – 'I should be able to do this, I'm so rubbish!'

As the sports psychiatrist Dr Steve Peters states:

> The word 'should' implies a standard or expectation. If you fail to reach that expectation then you have failed in your own world. The word 'should' is typically associated with such feelings as failure, blame, guilt, threat and inadequacy. All because we chose the word 'should'. If you had chosen the word 'could' then this does not evoke feelings of failure or set standards. Instead it is associated with feelings of opportunity, choice, possibility and hope. (Peters, 2012)

Once you start listening to your inner dialogue with curiosity, you can uncover the source of many of the challenges that you face. Consider the difference between 'I'd like to get this done by the end of the day', and 'I need to get this done by the end of the day'. One tiny word is probably all that lies between your being focused and getting it done, and watching yet another fascinating 'Business Insider' video online. Shifting from 'like' to 'want' to 'need' is a powerful management tool too.

You will have your own favourite inner-voice judgemental words. Once you become aware of them, you can start doing something about them and build your proactive resilience as a result.

What's your part in that?

When Fiona was training to be a life coach, she needed to gather a certain number of hours of sessions with clients, so I volunteered to be one.

At a very early stage, I ended up talking about a somewhat challenging relationship at work, where someone with a less than positive attitude would gradually spiral down into an increasingly negative mood as each day progressed.

Her question was quite simply: 'What's your part in their negative attitude?'

To my surprise, the little voice in my head reminded me that each day I would walk to my desk past theirs. As I was often privy to information from late-night teleconferences the previous day, I would share some of this information: 'You won't believe what happened last night when...'

It was as if I wanted to prod my colleague into a downward spiral, and, having been practising for several months, I had become quite expert in doing so.

The solution? Taking a different route to my desk, so I could not fan the flames so easily! Recognising the stories we are telling ourselves, and the part we are playing in what happens, can have a profound effect on our relationships.

Emotions versus mood

Turning to reactive resilience, we need to distinguish between emotions and mood. According to clinical psychologist Dr Pieter Rossouw: 'Emotions are different to mood, in that mood has a sustained rather than fleeting duration and it does not react to life events and environment.' (Rossouw, 2011)

While our emotions fluctuate due to what is happening (or has happened), our mood is more long term. Becoming more aware of both enables us to have more control, which in turn helps us feel better. It seems logical that the more we feel in control of situations, the better we feel. Research carried out by Kurt April and Kai Peters on locus of control showed that it is better to have a balance between feeling completely in control of events (an internal locus of control), and feeling that we have no influence over them (an external locus of control) (April and Peters, 2012). This is science showing us, as it has many times, that we need one another to be happy and successful.

Having a balance between a sense of internal and external control can also help us to have greater self-compassion. This in turn leads to a reduction in procrastination and stress, and an increase in happiness. We'll come back to it in Chapter 20.

Without awareness of our inner voice, we may say things that others find unhelpful or even hurtful, and later wonder why we said them at all. The animal voice is easy to recognise in all this, as it is likely to use words such as 'hard', 'unfair' or 'no one cares about me'. We need to learn to hear this and keep it under control.

You'll decorate the hedgerow

I often visit the Lake District on holiday: it is a great opportunity to try and get in some running training.

On a recent session, I was doing repetitions of a circuit with a short and steep uphill section. When I set out it was drizzling with rain, but it was only when I turned a corner that I discovered a biting, freezing headwind. Immediately my inner voice started up:

'This is too hard, let's stop!'
'Nope, we've got to do some laps and get some training in.'
'But this is hard work!' it screeched into my freezing ears.
After two laps I was actually feeling quite unwell, and after three I was positively nauseous, to the point at which I really thought I would be decorating the nearest hedge. Up starts the chatter again:
'I told you we should stop. We must stop. What will happen if you do throw up?'
'No one will see, and the rain will wash it away.'
'Let's stop, this is horrible!'
'Yes, it is horrible,' I countered. 'At the same time, it's making us work hard so we will become stronger, and that will improve how we get on in races. One more lap, OK?'
'Hmmmph. OK,' it replied.

I didn't decorate a hedgerow, and a warm shower soon restored normal body temperature. It would have been so easy to just give in at the first sign of the situation presenting a struggle.

Of course, sometimes things will go wrong. Being aware of our inner voice will provide us with a greater sense of control then, too. We need to focus *away* from the cause, and *towards* focusing on a useful response.

Gold medal crash

Elise Christie was the favourite for a gold medal representing Great Britain in the Winter Olympics 2018. Unfortunately, she was badly injured in a speed-skating heat. She still lined up for her next event, but tripped just off the line as the race started.

After a short delay the judges decided to restart the race, and she came second. Because of the earlier injury, which had been exacerbated by the crash, she had to be carried out.

As we were waiting for the official results, the news came through that she had been disqualified from the race. Having watched the whole story unfold over a couple of days, I expected to see a very angry and distressed interview.

To my, and everyone else's surprise, she calmly said: 'It is what it is... I'm going to...' Talk about self-control, awareness and dealing with inner dialogue. It will be interesting to see how her career unfolds from now on.

Next steps

1. Reflect on the last week. Think about what your inner voice has being saying that was helpful, and what was not (e.g. complaining).
2. How does your inner voice interfere when you are trying to cope in a tough situation? Write out the dialogue, then write an alternative, more empowering version.
3. Could you consider scheduling a daily check-in to notice your inner voice, and get it under control if need be?

7. Reframing

Put another way, it is not the event itself but the meaning we ascribe to it that makes the difference. The meaning is not a thing in itself but something we create in our mind, as we have explored already. The frame of reference is what we put around the meaning.

In any challenging situation where we are going to draw on our resilient capacity, it is important to adopt a solution-focus. One way to do this is to reframe the situation to explore alternative views, and find the most useful ones to employ. Therefore, reframing is a useful adaptive strategy – especially for building resilience.

Making meaning

What something means to you depends on a number of different aspects: the person creating the meaning, their knowledge, emotional state and the context and culture within which it happens. Meaning is truly a multifaceted thing, which you may never have thought of as being quite this complicated until now.

As a result of meaning coming from all these dimensions, the real meaning of an event is personally unique. We may share common phrases with which to describe them to others, but we all see them differently. Most importantly, when we change how we frame something, we alter the meaning that it has for us.

This does not mean ignoring the *actual* content of the event – it would be foolish to suggest otherwise; it just means changing how we feel about and react to it. We cannot change the past, as much as we would like to; but we can change what we do with it, which opens up new opportunities, perspectives and thus a greater sense of control. So reframing can change the future in a very real sense, as we will behave differently based on what we decide to learn from an event.

We can do this using a set of simple questions, illustrated here through an example of being unsuccessful in getting through a promotion board: 'I'm telling myself that I didn't get selected because my face doesn't fit.'

Q: What has to be true for the meaning you have made of this event to be valid?

A: *It is possible for a person to get selected. Someone else got selected instead of me.*

Q: What assumptions are contained within the story that you are telling yourself about this?

A: *There is a type of face that does fit, and I don't have it.*

Q: What beliefs and values do you have relating to this?

A: *People who have the right abilities should get promoted. Fairness is essential in all things. Nepotism is a bad thing.*

Q: How can I shift my perspective for this event to be useful to me?

A: *There is probably a better opportunity for me. This probably isn't the right role for me. If my face doesn't fit, then perhaps that is a sign that this isn't the right place for me anyway. Who did get selected? What can I learn from how they approached it? What could have gone better, and how can I change my preparation to make sure the same thing doesn't recur?*

Q: What is a positive result from this?

A: *I can stop worrying about promotion for another year, and get on with what I really want to do. I don't have the additional responsibility for another year, so I can use the time to learn something entirely new now.*

Q: When and/or where else might this experience be positive for you?

A: *When I go for any other kind of interviews, I'll now be better prepared.*

Obviously, your answers will be different for this event. It is unlikely that any one of these questions alone will change the meaning that you give to it, but applying them all will shake up your thinking because they change the frame you placed around it. Imagine that you are trying to get an old fence post out of the ground. You can dig around the base for a long time, but it still takes some wiggling backwards and forwards before it comes out completely.

This is a simplified version of a Neuro Linguistic Programming (NLP) model which I have found to be useful in my own life and when coaching others. If you are going to use it as presented here, make sure that you write the questions out first, leaving space to write your answers. Don't be tempted to type it all up as you go, as the process will be more enriching when done on paper with a pen or pencil. The insights you get will help you to decide possible action steps. It is always worthwhile talking them through with someone who has your best interests at heart, and committing to what you are going to do and when, as well as how much time you are going to give it.

While we have looked at this from a reactive resilient perspective, practising using the technique will be useful proactively as well. As the decorated Vietnam veteran and Vice-Admiral, James Stockdale, said:

> You must never confuse faith that you will prevail in the end – which you can never afford to lose – with the discipline to confront the most brutal facts of your current reality, whatever that may be. (Collins, 2001)

Next steps

1. Write out the reframing questions and your answers (or you can download a pre-printed sheet from: the-resilience-toolkit.com).
2. Make a plan for how you are going to move forward.

8. What is driving you?

'The TA [transactional analysis] concept of "drivers"... can generate a simple but compelling framework for analysing our characteristic styles of working.'

(Hay, 1996)

The five unconscious drivers

In 1975, clinical psychologist Taibi Kahler identified five unconscious drivers that motivate us, sometimes inappropriately, to satisfy our inner needs rather than reacting effectively to events. They were soon adopted as part of the core content of transactional analysis (Table 1).

Originally, these characteristics were presented as ways that we act in order to achieve approval from others, and used to understand how we operate when under stress – so understanding them is useful for both proactive and reactive resilience.

We have elements of each drive in our make-up, each with their own strengths and weaknesses. Table 1 shows them together with an example phrase that we might hear ourselves saying – either internally to ourselves, or out loud. They play out rather differently, as we shall soon see. (I have supplied additional definitions for ease of understanding.)

Driver (formal name)	Example phrases
Strength (Be strong)	I'm fine. Whatever happens, I'm not going to let you know what's going on for me. I can get through this, thanks.
Perfectionism (Be perfect)	This has to be absolutely right. It's not ready yet. OK, time's up.
Helpfulness (Please people)	I'm sorry. What can I do to help? Are you OK with everything?

Driver (formal name)	Example phrases
Persistence (Try hard)	I've got to try really hard. Going the extra mile is really important. Keep on keeping on.
Busyness (Hurry up)	I've got so much to do. I have to get this done now. Sorry I'm late.

Table 1: Five unconscious drivers in transactional analysis (based on Kahler, 1978)

It is important to note that while each has its own positive and negative aspects, it is possible for us to shift the mix between them. Let's look at each one in more detail.

Strength

People with a high strength driver ('Be strong') have an inner strength that is most obvious when in a crisis situation. When all around them is chaotic, they seem as calm as the proverbial cucumber. If you get to know them well, you may learn that inside they feel frantic and anxious, but they are thoroughly energised by such situations. Their apparent 'poker face' makes them great when negotiation is required too.

However, challenges come when things are difficult and they feel that they cannot turn to anyone else for help. Whether that is due to a lack of experience or knowledge, or just anxiety, this can create a lot of inner pressure – which, as we all know, has to leak out eventually.

Relying on their own resources to such a great extent can mean that novel problem situations leave them rather stuck. This driver can mean they find it hard to relax, sometimes leading to burnout because of a need to shoulder responsibilities in silence. As their manager, you may find it difficult to address performance and people-related issues with them, as they are so non-committal.

Imagine that you are in a meeting at work. Someone with a high strength driver will listen carefully, and speak when they are 100 per cent sure of themselves, but otherwise may remain very quiet. Sometimes this can mean that they will appear disinterested or even on edge. They will take away what they are asked to do, and ruminate on it and solve it alone. It is unlikely that you will hear any strong opinions expressed, but you will create a lot of discomfort if you press for such views during the meeting, or even afterwards during a one-to-one. However, if your meeting is caused by a critical issue, this is the person who will naturally assume leadership, directing the activities while appearing icy cool and calm.

If this is you, it is helpful to remind yourself that it is OK to share your feelings and show emotions – no one asked you to hang up your soul when you came to work, did they? It is OK to seek out help when you need it, and be real – this may be very important after being in a challenging situation, especially if it didn't go well. You might track the actual hours you are spending working, so that you can avoid getting burned out – and thus be ready when a crisis occurs.

Find something to do in your spare time that you enjoy and really stirs you, and make a personal commitment to do it. This will help you to connect with your emotions, and have a better awareness of what others might be feeling. Compare your level of this drive with the others, and look for where you could expand them as a way of building your resilience.

Perfectionism

People with a strong perfectionism driver ('Be perfect') create the very best work they possibly can. Their attention to detail is legendary. While others can let go of a draft document, someone with a high perfectionism driver finds that very difficult – you might have to prise it from their clenched hands! If you need a high degree of attention to detail and accuracy for contractual purposes, quality or performance inspections, they are your ideal person. If you cannot afford for something to go wrong, you need them on your team.

Challenges for people with this driver stem from their need to get everything right. Often they can end up being quite inefficient, consuming all the time and resources available. If given the opportunity, they will go on tweaking until they are forced to stop. They can be hard to please too, as their standards are higher than almost everyone else's. When timescales are tight, they need to work with others to set tight quality standards so that good enough is indeed good enough. Because of their need to drill into details, they find strategic, 'big-chunk' thinking difficult and potentially even dull.

In a meeting situation, someone with a high perfectionism driver will follow the usual business practices for successful meetings: i.e. a detailed agenda including timings, ensuring everyone has all the documents in advance, and logistics. During a meeting, they are the ones taking detailed notes and making sure that the agenda is adhered to by everyone. They want to know lots of detail around the things discussed and decisions made, and probably take a lot of the action themselves, especially if they feel that no one else can provide the necessary focus.

They may switch off if there is too much higher-level stuff going on, unless they can drill down into the details – others in the meeting may find this frustrating. When the minutes come out, probably at the last minute, they will be devastated if you find any errors.

If this describes you, it may help to set yourself more reasonable quality or performance standards, with a checklist against which to compare or validate. This will be useful in day-to-day activities, as well as when you face a crisis situation and have to make quick decisions (which otherwise you would find difficult). Give yourself shorter and firmer deadlines, and find someone you can trust who will gently hold you accountable to them. Working out what the true consequences of (what you see as) inaccuracies are, and letting other people know them when you point out errors, will be helpful to everyone involved.

Helpfulness

People with a high helpfulness driver ('Please people') are able to get along with pretty much anyone. They are incredibly helpful, easy-going and seem to have boundless capacity. Just the person you want in your team: they have an eye open for everyone else, and are acutely tuned to notice things that others don't, cutting them some slack if necessary. They are happy to take on plenty of tasks – that is, until they feel overburdened and unappreciated. Rather than say anything which might cause bad-feeling, they will just drop some tasks – and often the ones from which they themselves would benefit.

While the helpfulness driver is great in building relationships, people with this trait find challenging others difficult, and as a result can be seen as too sympathetic. They might struggle with decisions where others' needs are unclear, to the point of mind-reading them at times. Their ability to put others first can lead to burnout – which comes as a surprise to everyone involved, being unaware of all the things in progress. They can find leadership tough as a result of having to make difficult decisions and give challenging feedback.

In a meeting at work, a person with a high helpfulness driver will give a friendly welcome and thank everyone for attending; if they are leading it, they will agree an agenda through consultation. However, that agenda may not survive 'contact' for long, as they flex timings to ensure that everyone has their say. This can result in not achieving the purpose of the meeting; but as long as everyone is happy at the end, they will feel that they have done the right thing. When discussions become heated and tension rises, they will do what they can to defuse things and relieve discomfort. They will take a lot of the actions, especially if no one else steps forward, and may not challenge decisions if they feel that they are the only dissenting voice.

If you are like this, it will be useful to make as strong commitments with yourself as you are inclined to with others, so that you do not constantly work late, or on rest days or weekends. For example, this may mean making an arrangement to do something that you particularly enjoy after work with someone else. Trying to do less in this way will ready you for bringing your helpfulness to the fore, when faced with a really challenging situation in which you can make a significant difference.

It is important for you to work on recognising when you are extrapolating from a limited set of facts, and to avoid trying to read other people's minds, particularly in a crisis situation. The trick may be to ask more open-ended and richer questions. Lastly, telling others what you need, whether that is greater clarity or boundaries, will make a big difference to your resilience, and help to avoid burnout.

Persistence

People with a high persistence driver ('Try hard') always go the extra mile – whether that is staying late to complete tasks, or to have just one more go at getting something finished. It is as if they cannot put in anything less than 110 per cent in everything they do. They have a can-do attitude, which means they get stuck in and quickly get on with something new, looking at alternative ways of solving a problem or designing new processes. They are at their best when given clear criteria and autonomy for a task.

As you might expect, this persistence usually pays off, but at times they will put in more effort than is really necessary, sometimes resulting in a solution which is more complicated and takes longer than it might have done. As a result, they may never complete some tasks or projects, as there is always something else that they could do. This makes it really difficult when timescales are tight or when scope is not clearly defined. The word 'draft' is as much a challenge for these folk as for those driven by perfectionism.

In a meeting, a person with a strong persistence driver will arrive early, keen to get started. If appropriate, they will put forward lots of ideas and options, and will want to explore them in detail. This can leave other people slightly confused as to what decisions have been made, and what the next steps are. If they are leading, they need to make sure that all options are identified and explored, which can mean that the meeting overruns significantly, as multiple tangents are visited.

If you feel the need to be persistent in this way, it is worth ensuring that tasks have more clarity than you feel they really need, so that your work is well bounded. You might need to think more carefully before volunteering for everything – especially if it is new, and break tasks down to smaller and tighter time boxes, so that you have firmer deadlines within which to work. This might require finding a trusted accountability partner to keep you to your time boxes, and regularly evaluate your progress.

When crisis hits, your persistence is of great value – so long as you keep things as simple as possible. One way to achieve this is to imagine the route to a good outcome, and pursue that instead of trying to find the 'best' one. Proactively working on building your resilience through some of the other techniques in this book will help – but be sure to determine the boundaries first, of course!

Busyness

People with a strong busyness driver ('Hurry up') create a sense of speed around everything they do. This energy can get things started quickly and carry others along with it, driving hard towards deadlines. This is ideal where gaining initial momentum is required for either new or stalled tasks, and especially when situations are chaotic or in crisis. They naturally keep the main thing to the fore and are usually enthusiastic, seeing challenges as opportunities to learn, grow and make a difference.

It is quite common for someone to have 'Be busy' as a close or even same-scoring level as another driver, meaning that you get the best and worst of both. The downside of being so busy is mainly around timekeeping and paying sufficient attention to detail (much how James saw me, as described in the section on 'Inner maps'). They struggle to get things finished, and may get 85 per cent complete before moving on: it is as if the last 15 per cent bores them, and is not worth their focus. Many of us will be able to associate with this driver when we think about getting work done to a deadline: we think that we produce our best work under these situations, when actually research shows that while we complete it, it is not of as high quality as it could have been. It is worse than that though, because 'procrastinators end up suffering more and performing worse than other people' (Tice and Baumeister, 1997).

Sometimes, this need for speed will see standard operating procedures ignored or bypassed in a drive to resolve a situation. At its extreme, the sheer whirlwind of this speed-driven type can leave others trailing in their wake, wondering what just hit them. They are great to have in your team when you need to get moving, but they do need encouragement to be punctual, and slow down a little to keep everyone else with them.

In a meeting at work, the person with a high busyness driver is easy to identify, as they are not there: they will rush in late, apologising profusely that their last appointment overran. Often they will not have read the necessary paperwork, and thus slow things down while you explain it. With their mind running at a million miles an hour, they think they have understood what is being discussed before actually hearing the whole story.

If this describes you, is it time to slow down a bit? Think about how you might be able to plan your time (see the section in Part 3 on effectiveness), as at your velocity, burnout could be just around the corner – never mind the burn marks that you are leaving behind you as you sprint from one thing to another!

Avoiding overwork can make you prepared for when workload escalates rapidly due to a crisis. Break things down, and visualise how you want them to be when you have finished. Use that detail to plan each day, leave more margin than you might normally have done, and set yourself some personal milestones. Try to really listen to what is being said at meetings, and pause rather than talking over others. You might find it helpful to explore a simple mindfulness practice, as it will make your days calmer and build your resilience for when times are really tough.

Next steps

1. You can download a summary sheet including a pen-portrait and questionnaire of each driver at: the-resilience-toolkit.com
2. Talk to someone you can trust to get a perspective on how you show up in both proactive and reactive situations.
3. Decide which driver you are going to work on increasing, and build a plan. Get some coaching if your drivers cause you significant challenges with burnout.

9. Temperament

> 'There are two sides to personality, one of which is temperament and the other character. Temperament is a configuration of inclinations, while character is a configuration of habits. Character is disposition, temperament pre-disposition.'
>
> (Keirsey, 1998)

David Keirsey was so fascinated with what made people act as they do that he made it his life's work. In essence he says that at our core, we have some built-in attributes that life experience moderates to produce our character. While our experience continues to build day by day, our core temperament remains the same.

Temperament theory, as researched and validated by Keirsey, assigns meaningful descriptions to each of four groups based on two easily observed factors:

- How people communicate – whether they talk about facts and specific information (which he labelled 'Concrete'), or about ideas, theories and general information ('Abstract').
- How people choose and use tools – following a set of rules or norms (which he termed 'Cooperative'), or doing what works, adopting and adapting, sometimes disregarding the norms ('Utilitarian').

Table 2 on the next page shows the core characteristics of each.

- Concrete Utilitarians have an 'Artisan' temperament, with a natural strength in tactical action (the 'Just do it' type of person).
- Concrete Cooperatives are described as having a 'Guardian' temperament, with a natural strength in logistical activities (the 'Mind the shop' kind of person).
- Abstract Cooperative is the 'Idealist' temperament, with a natural ability in diplomacy (the encouraging, 'I know you can' type).
- Abstract Utilitarians are described as having a 'Rational' temperament, with a natural ability for strategic thinking and action (the 'Hmm now, let's see' type).

	Abstract communication	**Concrete communication**
Cooperative working	Idealist temperament • Seeks meaning and relationships • Personal identity • Intuitive • Enthusiastic • Uniqueness • Influencer • Future-oriented • Emotive • Prefers to work with people	Guardian temperament • Seeks security and stability • Dependable • Loyal • Desires consistency • Conserving • Responsible • Cautious • Orderly • Industrious
Utilitarian working	Rational temperament • Intellectual • Logical • Future-oriented • Problem-solver and persistent • Ingenious • Desires knowledge • Values competency • Open-minded • Precise	Artisan temperament • Enjoys freedom • Exciting • Thrill-seeker • Optimistic and cheerful • Works best in a crisis • Thrives on impulse • Seeks variety • Determined • Courageous

Table 2: Core characteristics of temperament theory
Source: Keirsey (1998)

You probably have skills across many of the quadrants. Temperament theory is about *what comes most naturally to you* – how you would like to be if you were unfettered by the expectations and even the 'rules' imposed on you by others.

The key thing is, we are all different. We all experience the world differently, and we can all learn. Of course, with sufficient experience it is perfectly possible for someone with, say, an Artisan temperament, to be organised in the way that someone with a Guardian temperament is – but it will not be as natural or effortless. This can lead to stress and burnout if pursued for too long.

Here, we are after useful *insights* more than *absolutes*. I have used the Keirsey Temperament Sorter (KTS-ii) toolset for more than 10 years with a variety of teams and individuals, and it never fails to provide new viewpoints and trigger valuable conversations around what is going on for them. Of course no profiling tool is 100 per cent accurate – humans are far too complex to be described through any model – but the KTS-ii has proved itself to be more useful than other similar tools, especially for teams.

Let's take a look at each in turn to see how they might shape our resilience.

The four temperaments according to Keirsey

Artisan temperament

If, like me, you have an Artisan temperament, then you do what works and deal with what you find in front of you.

Building your resilience is anathema to you, as you are much more reactive than proactive. You make an excellent champion for development activities, especially when paired with someone of Idealist temperament who you get on with – just be aware that with the difference between you in how you use words, tools and techniques, both of you may have to choose carefully.

You are well placed to do any training or delivery necessary, enjoying the spotlight. You might not like creating the materials as much, and with diplomacy as your lowest strength, need to be careful how you come across to others at times.

'Crisis' is almost your middle name. Not that you create it, but you thrive in fast-paced situations that are exciting for you: these are where you really come alive. Quick on your feet, excited by the cut-and-thrust, it is important for you to be aware that while tactical thinking is your main strength, strategy is lower, and diplomacy lowest of all.

So do the 'what' thinking with your colleagues of a Rational temperament, and the 'how' thinking yourself. Hand over as much of the communications necessary to someone with an Idealist temperament, and draw on the innate logistical skills of your Guardian temperament teammates to get the right equipment in place. When it is all over, take time out to properly rest, and reflect together with everyone else on what you can learn and implement for the future.

Guardian temperament

With a Guardian temperament, you are drawn to facts and what is, and you do what is expected. Having standard operating procedures in place can help you with both building your resilience proactively, and maintaining a resilient approach reactively.

Where there are processes established, you will happily follow them to build your resilience. The challenge comes when it is up to you to decide, so you should consider making time to agree what is expected of you. You find it easy to live out what has been agreed and demonstrate it in practice, which also helps those reporting to you to do the same. No 1.30 am emails from you!

With strategy as your weakest suit, the best thing would be to find someone with a Rational temperament to help you think through the bigger picture. With your drive for facts, you may find it hard to come up with ideas for proactive resilience building – in which case, seek out a friendly Idealist temperament colleague, as they will bring a tad more humanity to your thinking (not because you overlook others, just that considering their view is a little more difficult for you than Idealist temperament folk).

In a crisis, you will follow established protocols and procedures to the letter. While that is always going to be helpful, when things start to go outside 'normal' boundaries, you may find it harder to improvise. Turn, then, to an Artisan temperament colleague, who is naturally gifted in such situations. You will bring a calm orderliness to challenging times, as your natural strength with logistics comes to the fore. You may need to be a touch more flexible in what gets used for what, and abandon the checklists that you love.

Idealist temperament

If you have an Idealist temperament then you are interested and naturally think in terms of what could be, while also following rules and procedures as defined.

When thinking about growing resilience, you naturally want to include other people and provide for them. You are gifted in building relationships and helping others to do so, which can provide a foundation for both your and their resilience when challenges arise. Your enthusiastic nature can help others to really engage with activities and training aimed at building resilience, and you make an excellent champion for them. The challenge might be for you to work as hard at building your own resilience, as well as that of others.

In tough situations, while you face similar challenges to those with a Guardian temperament, your intuitive sense of what is going on for others around you can be invaluable. Your sense of the emotions involved in a situation can cause you to burn a lot of emotional energy if a situation is particularly upsetting. In this case, you may need the support of someone of a Rational temperament to take a more objective viewpoint.

The fact that you are future-oriented by nature gives you the strength to focus on solutions in the moment, rather than getting stuck in analysis paralysis of the 'Why did this happen' kind. When things are back under control, you will have time to evaluate and learn from what happened for the future, which naturally you will want to share with others.

Rational temperament

If you have a Rational temperament, you naturally think in terms of strategy, doing what works with what is available to hand, while considering ideas and what could be.

To build your resilience, you will have a strategy or want one to be in place. What you come up with may be hard for others to understand, especially your Guardian colleagues, in which case you might want to develop it jointly rather than alone. As logical thinking is part of your make-up, what you come up with will make perfect sense to you, particularly in considering future eventualities. Other people might not find it so clear, however.

The challenge will come from having lesser skills in arranging the nuts and bolts required, and perhaps more fundamentally, carrying others with you. In this case, engage with your Artisan and/or Idealist temperament colleagues to do that with you.

When disaster does strike, much as you would hope it wouldn't, your cool, calm and strategic thinking means that you are not inclined to just try something and see what happens. This makes you well placed to take overall command of the situation. However, you will need to maintain your focus on what needs to be done, rather than how to do it – which needs a more concrete set of thinking skills and therefore better suited to those of a Guardian or Artisan temperament.

Guardians are great for getting the right kit where it needs to be, and checking that procedures are followed correctly; while Artisans are best suited to get stuck in and just make things happen through their adaptable nature – something that you will appreciate, as you share that with them. Although you are good at problem-solving, it is from a more logical perspective rather than a practical one – so again, reach out to an Artisan to work with you.

Next steps

1. Find out your temperament by visiting: keirsey.com
2. Build an action plan for working on both your proactive as well as your reactive resilience, using temperament as a lens.
3. Consider your teammates' and stakeholders' temperaments, and think about how you might work together better.
4. Grab a summary and pen-portrait for each temperament at: the-resilience-toolkit.com

10. Mindset and motivation

'The way we get feedback on our performance in life can fundamentally limit or expand our future achievements.'

(Dr Carol Dweck, 2006)

In every team and walk of life, we come across people who are willing to go the extra mile, as well as those who are not. In a recent workshop I led, one participant described this challenge as: 'Is it "wants to but can't", or "can do but won't"?'

Often we put lack of motivation down to deliberate belligerence. But what if it isn't? What if there is something else at play? One of the key contributors seems to be the mindset that we hold.

Psychologist Carol Dweck carried out research which found that on the one hand, by praising ability ('I can see you're really good at this'), a person's performance tends to plateau: on the principle of 'If I'm good at something, then I don't need to try hard because it's a natural gift. I can't build my capacity or ability. If it's something I'm not naturally gifted at, there's no beating nature.' This she labelled as a 'fixed mindset'.

Dweck found that, on the other hand, by praising effort or process ('I can see you tried really hard'), recipients' performance tends to build: on the principle that 'I know I can work hard, and I can learn how to do things that are more challenging. Whatever happens, I'm sure that I can at least *try* hard.' This she labelled as a 'growth mindset'.

While the research was applied initially within an educational context, it is now making in-roads into organisations. The details are beyond the scope of this book, but you can easily read about them in her book *Mindset: The New Psychology of Success* (2006).

> ### You don't have the language gene
>
> As a child finding learning French difficult, I remember being told: 'It's your father who is the linguist in this family, I don't think you inherited his ability.'

> This was what was commonly believed at the time – rather than being a deliberate intention to limit my performance, which is what it did.

With a fixed mindset, you have a belief that limits your performance. You may find other people's success as personally challenging, and might even go so far as to minimise or undermine their achievements. When things do go wrong, you readily point to a cause that lies outside you or your control (you may remember sports personalities who behaved like that in the past). Faced with a crisis situation, a fixed mindset can result in feeling disempowered and stuck, hence more stress than you really need to have.

A growth mindset is more expansive and liberating. When things don't go as well as you had hoped, you frame it as opportunity to learn – either from the experience itself, or from someone else who has been successful in the same situation. You delight in others' achievements and success. You are willing to have a go at new things when the opportunity arises, and when faced with a challenging situation, your resilience is naturally higher – not that you don't find it stressful, but you naturally reframe it to be a learning opportunity, knowing that it will pass.

	Fixed mindset	Growth mindset
Challenges?	Avoid	Embrace
Obstacles?	Give up	Persist
Effort?	Pointless	The path to mastery
Feedback?	Worthless	Priceless
Others success?	A threat	Opportunity to learn
End result =	Performance plateaus to mediocrity	Performance builds to mastery

Our mindset is probably more of a continuum than strong polarisation either way. It is important to be aware that we are all a mix of both mindsets: in some contexts we will have a growth mindset, whereas in others we may be more fixed. Of course, there will be times in life – whether through stress or illness – when even with a strong growth mindset the very best that we can do is put one foot in front of the other, and get to the end of the day – which can look very fixed mindset. At least we give it our best, even if 'best' isn't particularly good.

Encouraging the shift: a growth mindset formula

How can we shift towards more of a growth mindset, and propel our team's performance upward? The way I express it is through this simple formula:

Challenge + Determination + Effort + Feedback = Growth

As this shows, the steps to move towards a more growth mindset approach are:

1. Setting an appropriate challenge – one that requires a good amount of stretch, without being out of bounds for the individual or team concerned. One that is motivating.
2. Encouraging a high level of grit and/or determination.
3. Applying a high degree of effort over an extended period of time.
4. Getting (or giving) valuable, actionable feedback – probably the most important aspect of this formula (which we shall return to in Part 4).

For reactive resilience building, having a growth mindset means that you see opportunities to grow through the trials and tribulations that you encounter, even if you don't do it brilliantly well to start with – and naturally, you will be seeking out someone from whom you can learn.

A more fixed mindset sees you thinking that you cannot do what is required, that you are out of your depth or beyond your abilities. Choose to counter this inner dialogue, set yourself an achievable interim challenge – one to which you are willing to apply consistent effort and determination. Then, despite all your misgivings, get someone to give you some well-crafted, grounded and actionable feedback.

Motivation

In *Drive*, Daniel Pink explores the various facets of motivation. In particular, he describes the progression of this key leadership skill. The first motivational approach was about basic survival needs, i.e. the motivation to gather food, have shelter and ensure the survivability of the species.

The second approach added the 'carrot and stick' method. This was driven by thinkers such as the mechanical engineer Frederick Winslow Taylor, who was interested in increasing factory worker productivity. He created the concept of seeing people as machines or part of a machine: to get them to perform better, you reward people for doing what you want, and punish the behaviour that you don't. Many organisations still apply only these techniques, sadly. The problem is that rewards such as profit-related-pay cease to work over time, as they just become 'part of the package'.

The third motivational approach (Pink says) is one that provides tasks that enable people to build mastery, autonomy and purpose. Thus motivation comes from within, and has intrinsic benefits such as personal success, rather than extrinsic ones such as money or fame.

Cash as a catalyst

As the father of two teenagers, I am already hearing the discussions that they and their peers are having about their careers. It is never about making a lot of money, but more often about doing something that aligns with who they are, and what they find interesting and absorbing.

More significantly, they don't talk about careers as long term or with big earning potential or bonuses. They are interested in doing work that has a clear purpose: being sustainable, and for the greater good. Cash is a catalyst, not an objective, for them.

The results of being purpose-focused in this way can reduce burnout, exhaustion, anxiety and to some level, depression.

Find any interview with a world-class musician such as Yehudi Menuhin, and you will notice that when asked if they have achieved mastery, they say things like: 'I shall never achieve mastery, it's a constant journey to playing better.' This is about iterative improvement, which arises through having engaging work and a growth mindset as well as regular and actionable feedback. It results in increased satisfaction, productivity and achievement, and reduced anxiety, boredom and frustration.

Micromanagement be gone

When I joined Hewlett-Packard in 1996, the founders were still alive, and we could all get a copy of *The HP Way* (1995) by Bill Hewlett and David Packard.

Two of Packard's principles really stood out for me then, and still do today: 'People don't come to work to do a bad job.' The second one was something like 'Keep the tools unlocked, allow people to work where and when they need to' – showing just how far ahead of the curve he and Hewlett were in their leadership thinking.

People are more motivated when they get to choose how – and to some extent, as the task or job provides, where, when and with whom – they work. Micromanagement be gone. The results of such radical thinking is that processes, performance and retention increase, while burnout and stress decrease. This is closely coupled to building resilience.

Those of us brought up to use the second type of motivation would do well to understand and make the necessary shifts quickly to the third type, if we are to engage with the next generation – especially if we are to do so in a way to build their resilience.

If all we do is praise people for being good at or suited for their job, then we should not be surprised if they decline more challenging tasks in the future. When we praise them for their effort, it will be a completely different story.

Next steps
1. Find out your mindset by going to:
   blog.mindsetworks.com/what-s-my-mindset
2. What could be a useful first step to take to improve your resilience by applying growth mindset principles?
3. Decide one area in which you would like to build your resilience, and try applying the growth mindset formula.

11. Attitude and adversity

> 'When we are no longer able to change a situation, we are challenged to change ourselves… Everything can be taken from a man but one thing: the last of the human freedoms – to choose one's attitude in any given set of circumstances, to choose one's own way.'
>
> (Frankl, 2004)

Attitude

As we saw in the Introduction, coping strategies include an element of being able to change our emotional reaction to what is happening around us. Regulating our emotions is not about *not* feeling things, but about controlling how we respond to them – just like life experiences, it is what you do with them that counts.

As we saw when considering inner voice (Chapter 6), emotions are the language of the animal brain and are an offer, not an instruction – we always have a choice in how to respond, rather than allowing our emotions to drive behaviours blindly.

Shifting our emotional response may lead to a sense of having less control over a situation. Therefore, it is important to:

- acknowledge the emotions
- consider their origin
- accept responsibility or blame
- exercise some self-control
- take an appreciative stance, by considering what is good about it and how we might increase positive elements
- choose and adapt a more useful reaction – our emotions usually change when we find valid reasons for them.

The benefits of managing our emotions are covered extensively in emotional intelligence literature and are beyond the scope of this book, so I will not revisit that ground here. However, it is worth remembering that those folk who are not good at managing their emotions are often exhausting and stressful for those around them, and harder to work with due to their unpredictable nature. If anyone ever says 'I never know how they're going to show up', that should be a significant red flag to you. As psychotherapist and organisational consultant Shane Warren

(2013) states: 'Society is defined by the way in which social interchanges are co-ordinated. Healthy societies require the individuals within them to regulate how emotions are experienced and expressed.'

People often use their emotional state as an internal indicator of their capabilities and, in turn, to drive their behaviour.

Expending energy can create more

When training for the London Marathon, there were days when I would get home from work, tired and somewhat stressed. Finding a long training run in the plan, I would have to really steel myself to get out into the darkness, wondering if I would be able to complete the session.

I soon learned that my feeling of exhaustion was not the same as the physical state brought on by a hard workout – in fact, I often returned home from training feeling that I would have more energy than when I had set out. Emotions can be fickle things, but they are not always wrong.

It can be helpful to separate difficult events into either challenges or threats.

- Challenges are difficult tasks and life experiences where we have sufficient resources to meet the demands placed on us.
- Threats are those where the resources we have are insufficient.

Threats elevate our stress hormones, with resulting negative health consequences; whereas challenges may not. Notice the connection here to reframing (which we looked at earlier in Chapter 7).

In 'Managing at the speed of change' Daryl Conner describes a continuum of resilience, from type-D (low resilience) – who experience the world as right/wrong, good/bad and life as generally punishing – to type-O (high resilience) – interpreting the world as multifaceted and generally rewarding.

Clearly, how we think, and what we believe about a situation influences how we behave when we find ourselves in tough times:

- how well we can control our situation
- the level of effort we choose to apply to either coping with it, or resolving it

- our level of perseverance
- how vulnerable we are to stress and depression.

It therefore makes sense to evaluate these and choose to adopt and/or develop more useful beliefs.

It is also useful to build our abilities to learn, as research by Wheatley in 2011 found that people with stronger abilities to learn tend to treat problems and difficulties as challenges rather than as threats. Conversely, those who have lower self-belief about their ability to learn tended to treat these as threatening situations. Notice the link here to having a growth mindset: if you believe that you can learn, you are more likely to evaluate a situation as a challenge rather than a threat.

People who have high self-efficacy see difficult tasks as challenges to be mastered, as opposed to threats to avoid. As a result, they define challenging goals to which they are strongly committed, with that commitment increasing even when things do not go well. When that happens, they see the apparent failure as due to insufficient effort, knowledge or skills. They also approach threatening situations with confidence, whereas those who have lower levels of self-belief pull back from difficult tasks, viewing them as a potential threat.

Practising gratitude

Considering our blessings has come to be part of mindfulness practice. Whether that is practising 'an attitude of gratitude', or the more old-fashioned 'counting your blessings', this has been proven to be beneficial – especially when they have strong personal meaning.

It can be useful to consider as a resilience practice in challenging times, as it enables us to step back from the melee.

Adversity

'Life is a whirling torrent for which nobody has a script.'

(Poynton, 2008)

At some level, this entire book could be considered as being about this single idea. The aim here is to give you a way of thinking through and dealing with adversity, so that you feel more resilient when you think it may happen, and so that you have a way of thinking about it when it does.

Change, and the adversity often accompanying it, is a natural feature of life. Yet the deep roots of our animal brains seek consistency and tend towards being controlling. So when things do not go as we planned or desired, we can experience feelings of failure, embarrassment and even shame.

Facing up to this fact is essential, if we are to be more resilient in the face of adversity. There are three phases that can be useful to transition through: acknowledgement, acceptance and action.

Acknowledgement

In every situation there are known and unknown elements, so they are not straightforward. Especially where there are people involved, and when nothing is uncomplicated! It is important that we acknowledge the true reality of a situation: something has either gone wrong, or not as well as it might have. It may not be wholly our fault, but either way, something needs to be done.

The first step to consider is the event: what part of it, and how much, is actually down to you alone? Not the situation, context or environment – just your bit. Ask yourself:

- What did I intend?
- Did I do my best?
- Could the situation have been anticipated?
- What part did anyone else play?

The point is to be realistic about what happened. If it was truly not down to you, then you can move on to the next step.

What really matters is that we are honest with ourselves about what happened, so that we can learn from it and act differently next time.

One great way of ensuring that is to review an event soon after its occurrence, and pause at each point where you made a decision. For each one, identify in detail some alternative decisions that could have been more useful. Then, choose which one would be best to apply next time. The result will be that when the situation recurs, you will be more resourceful. Better still, it will give you something to draw on, even if the situation is slightly different.

Acceptance

We need to accept that we are not perfect, and that we are unable to control everything. As we saw in Chapter 6, the challenge we face is the inner tension between the human and animal parts of our brain. We might need to remind ourselves that despite all our best efforts, perfection is not possible. Indeed, a lot of the time it actually can be undesirable.

Of course, this is not about just shrugging it off. Still, whether you have to face the fact that everyone misses a target sometimes, or that what happened was not all down to you – accepting that we are all flawed, and being gracious with ourselves (and others), is the fastest way to move forward.

> 'We must make the best use that we can of the things that are in our power, and use the rest according to their nature.'
>
> Epictetus

Action

First, breathe! When we are under pressure, we often start to breathe more rapidly, and therefore from the top of our lungs. As a result there is a residual amount of CO_2 in the bottom that is not exhaled. This can trigger an increase in breathing rate, which just increases residual CO_2. To stop the cycle, we need to pause and breathe deeply, even if only for 30 seconds. (I have found this to work during times of increased anxiety, such as dealing with late trains!)

While it would be unhelpful to totally ignore what went wrong, it is important to switch to a solution-focused attitude as quickly as possible. After all, there is not much we can do about it now that it has happened, so we might as well look at how we can move forward. (Obviously, a lot of that depends on the details of the situation. It is most definitely not about working out how to hide or deflect attention.)

Next steps

1. Which step in the acknowledge–acceptance–action process do you think is the greatest challenge for you?
2. Think about what your key drivers are, and the impact that your temperament has on each one. What could be a small initial step to take the next time you are facing a difficult situation?

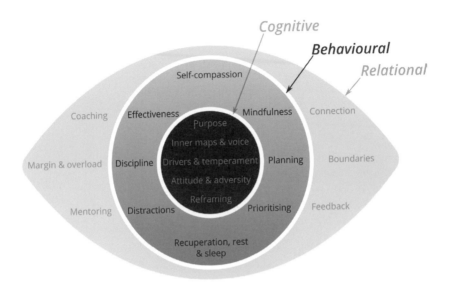

Part 3: Behavioural factors

12. Peak effectiveness times

Tracking your effectiveness

Many of us believe we are 'morning people' or 'night owls'. As always, what we believe becomes our reality. But how do you really *know* that? Unless we have actually done some investigation, we do not have any evidence. Knowing your peak effectiveness times (PETs) can help you plan what to do when. It's easy to find out – here are some practical ideas.

Figure 6 is an example of how to track your PETs.

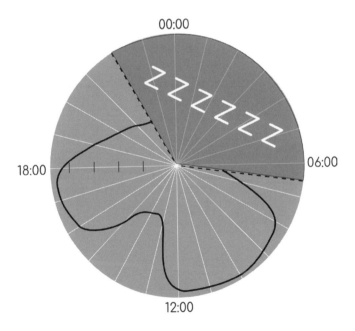

Figure 6: Peak effectiveness time monitor

Start off by shading out the hours you spend asleep – marked 'ZZZ' in this case. Once you have this in place as a starting point, the rest is simply a matter of doing an hourly check-in.

Start by tracking your effectiveness level. With a score of 1 at the centre of the chart, and 5 at the outer edge, you can see that I have found mine to be low – 2 out of 5 until around 8.30 am, rising to 4–5 until around 12.30 pm, when it drops quite dramatically. It rises again around 3 pm, until at 4 pm when I am firing on all cylinders again. This lasts for a couple of hours, then drops steadily until 10 pm.

Armed with this data, I have changed my approach to what type of work I do and when:

- Plan the day from 8–8.30 am (including prayer and reading time).
- Deep work requiring concentration and focus for 90-minute periods, with short breaks between them until 12.30 pm.
- Lunch followed by admin tasks such as email, finances, etc. until 3 pm.
- Creative thinking-type work until 5.30 pm, when I typically review the day's progress before ending at 6–7 pm.

Your day will not be the same, but this gives you some idea of how to use the data you gather. You'll notice from the above list that I do not deal with email before 12 pm, nor coffee meetings. Why would I give away my most focused working time to something trivial? Of course, if someone is willing to pay for my services, then they get what they ask for!

A word or two about deep work – the label given by Cal Newport in his book of the same name to the type of concentrated, focused, deliberate work, as opposed to shallow work – which we need for working with large amounts of material such as legislation or writing detailed reports.

Newport says that the younger generation are less able to do work of this nature, because one of the key requirements is to avoid task switching – which as we shall see later, significantly reduces our ability to concentrate. For now, just note that switching compromises deep work. If that type of work is what your job requires, and you feel the weight of tasks that seem to never make any progress, this may be the reason.

When you take it to the next stage and map your motivation and energy levels, you will be able to decide things such as when it is better to work on particular types of task (including those that you are not very interested in) and when it is best to exercise or have some 'down time'.

Mapping your PETs is the only way that you are going to know for certain if you are a lark, an owl or 'third bird' as Daniel Pink (2018) describes them – someone who falls between the two. Once you have the data, then you can plan which tasks are best suited for you to do and when. If you lead a team, it can be extremely valuable to have everyone do the same analysis, and overlay the results. You might decide to make some significant changes as a result.

Why's the meeting then?

I covered this topic with a legal firm that I once worked with: 80 per cent of them decided that they should be doing case work between 8 am and 12 pm, yet slap-bang in the middle of that was a 9.15 am team meeting. A partner in the room bravely confessed that this time had been chosen to make everyone come in on time.

When we mapped the whole team's PETs on a flip chart, they quickly decided that the best time for their team meeting was 1.30 pm. The result was that they were able to get more of the concentrated – deep – work done in the morning, which was the most effective time for the majority of them.

It is not always going to be possible to get everyone to move their meetings in this way, of course – especially if you are the only owl or third bird. The key is that you now have some information that not only enables you to maximise your effectiveness but – and maybe more importantly – also understand why certain activities are a greater challenge for you at certain times of day.

If, for example, you become involved in a situation that requires you to work extended hours, or on a high-pressure project, and this in turn means that you are having to be on your 'A-game' for an extended period, now you understand why you become overly tired or stressed.

One of the key things to build your resilience is planning and taking recuperation time (as we shall see later). If you anticipate a challenging time ahead, you can plan in recuperation beforehand as well. Knowledge of your PETs means that you already know when it is best for you to rest as well.

> ### Plan around your non-PETs
>
> I often end up travelling away from home to run workshops in different places. One of those was recently to deliver a keynote speech in Newport, South Wales in the afternoon, followed by a 3 hr 30 min drive to Chesterfield at a dinner with the regional superintendents' association, then deliver a workshop to them the next morning before driving home.
>
> Knowing my PETs, and how much energy this type of work takes from me, I planned a quieter day beforehand and arranged to break the return journey at a friend's home, as well as planning in a few hours of recovery time the following day.

Once you know your PETs and start using them for deep work, just watch how much you get done!

Timing decisions

> 'Afternoons are the Bermuda triangle of our days.'
>
> (Pink, 2018)

Having understood more about ourselves, there are some other general principles that are useful to understand. I have placed this section purposefully after you have done the research, so that you do not have to just accept or reject what I am about to share!

Our internal body clock creates a rhythm that influences all the elements of our bodies and minds – the circadian rhythm. As a result, most of us are better at doing focused, detailed work in the mornings, and creative tasks in the afternoons. The mornings are better for focused work because we have the greatest stores of willpower then. As willpower is depleted, we become worse and worse at controlling our impulses.

Creative thinking improves during the afternoon, because thinking outside the box requires that we relinquish some of our normal inhibitions. So, the best time to perform a specific task depends on the nature of that task – as we have already established.

To ensure that we make good decisions in the afternoons, it is worth working with a team that comprises people with a more owl-like rhythm – which makes it even more important to know when our PETs are. Better still, to sleep on the decision until the following morning.

It is possible to remotivate ourselves somewhat after energy depletion. While we are all different (you will need to experiment for yourself), some people find exercise or just a sociable lunchtime (rather than one trying to catch up on email or social media) can be helpful.

Use lunchtimes to have a clear break to get away from your desk, hang out with colleagues with no particular purpose in mind, and preferably get some fresh air. Even a short walk has been shown to have beneficial effects on our stress levels and mental health. You cannot work in-depth for more than a couple of hours, so listen to what your body is telling you and take a break!

From the perspective of personal organisation, you might find it useful to re-plan the rest of the day, setting shorter timescales and making commitments based on a renewed vision of who you are performing a task for, and how they will benefit. Notice that there is a definite sense of looking forward here.

A beautiful wake

One holiday when I was a teenager, we went to Spain. In the garage of our villa there was a Topper dinghy. As a keen sailor, I quickly got it out on the water, released from the shackles of an overly hot beach, zipping across the waves.

With a stable current and a healthy breeze, I turned to admire my own wake, proud to see the evidence of my boat-handling skills. Until, that is, I noticed my feet getting wet. Turning to look forward, I found that the nose of the dinghy was ploughing into the waves, with the sea pouring in.

The wake you leave may be beautiful, but if you only consider what is behind you and what you have done, you will stall and may get a nasty surprise.

To avoid dips in drive, enthusiasm and energy in the first place, try taking a leaf out of former US President Barack Obama's book by avoiding having to use willpower unnecessarily, early in the day. In his case this meant having suits and shirts pressed and ready, so that choosing what to wear did not drain this precious resource.

Beginning well should include being clear on the outcomes that you hope to achieve, and the benefits to yourself and others, as this will give you the opportunity to create some initial momentum.

Anticipating the obstacles that may cross your path will reduce their energy-sapping impact too – perhaps through the use of a pre-mortem technique (i.e. imagining that you're at the end of the day and that it has been an unmitigated disaster, before considering what happened to make it that way). Creating some milestones in your day to pause, take stock and make some course corrections before continuing on can help. These landmarks can 'shake us out of the tree so we can glimpse the forest' (Pink, 2018).

Thinking about this from a proactive resilience stance, it is clear that we need to do some self-discovery while we are away from a heated situation. Knowing when our energy dips – and more importantly, what can restore that energy, even if only slightly – can help us to build plans for when we are placed in challenging situations at suboptimal times of day.

You will now be aware that you might make poorer decisions at the end of the day, or a long shift, in times of trial. As far as possible, use the procedures and/or checklists that you have created – whether they are your organisation's standard operating procedures, or just personal ones – and if you can, triangulate the decisions with other people who are less tired or more of a night-owl temperament.

When you are in a crisis situation, try to do focused work in the morning, and take more breaks when you physically extricate yourself to recharge. Stopping, stepping back, breathing and taking deliberate action while remembering who you are doing it for – all of this will help you maintain resilience until the storm passes.

Next steps

1. Are you a lark, owl or third bird? How do you know? Plot your effectiveness for the next week or two to really find out. Go to the-resilience-toolkit.com to get a blank PET map.
2. What is best, and when? Can you move things, or at least plan differently?
3. What about the team you lead or are part of? Encourage them to find their PETs too. Use what you discover to move things such as team meetings and one-to-ones.

> 'Discipline isn't a dirty word. Far from it. Discipline is the one thing that separates us from chaos and anarchy. Discipline implies timing. It's the precursor to good behaviour, and it never comes from bad behaviour. People who associate discipline with punishment are wrong: with discipline, punishment is unnecessary.'
>
> Brannaman

Discipline

While the word 'discipline' has fallen out of fashion because of the overtones of being controlled by another or punishment, the fact is: *discipline sets you free.*

While this quote could be about physical discipline, which does have its place in building resilience (as we will see later), here we are more interested in having a consistent approach to what we do in life.

Many people respond to this idea with something along the lines of 'I don't want to be highly organised in my own life, it's bad enough having a boss breathing down my neck all week – at the weekend I want space and freedom to do what I feel like!' – and amen to that. Balance is important. Downtime and real rest is important – although I think many of us don't know how to do that any more either. Never mind dealing with the challenge of a micromanaging boss... that definitely takes resilience!

Where does this idea come from that a good life is one where we just go with the flow? Surely a good life is one that is lived on purpose: with a bigger aim in mind? We know intuitively that the only way we are going to succeed at a complex goal is by consistent, aligned action towards it. Sounds just like discipline, doesn't it?

Discipline avoids disaster

When I decided to run the London Marathon, I started to take my training very seriously. Not just because it is a physically tough challenge, but because I wanted to set a time that would guarantee me entry to the race the following year: the target time was 2:45. I found

---

a training plan, learned about how it worked, adapted it for me, and then stuck to it absolutely without fail – except when I was unable to, due to illness.

That meant lovely runs through the autumn forests and fields with friends, which was easy. It also meant 10-mile runs after work in the depths of winter rain and wind, which was horrible. And 22-mile-long, slow distance run with the lads, which often had us weeping with pain and exhaustion at the end.

Not surprisingly, the results came eventually, although it seemed at times that there was little improvement. My half-marathon time came down from 1:30 to 1:14. My 10-mile time dropped to 54 minutes, and 10k to 34 minutes (and my only race win).

The discipline of daily training made all the difference over time, and prepared me well for the rigours ahead. But six days before the event, I got food poisoning and ended up in bed for two days. A quick time trial showed that my mile time was still under six minutes. On the day I finished in 2:51:23 – all because of a year of discipline and focus.

I can imagine you nodding in agreement. It's a no-brainer: if you want to do well at a sporting event such as the marathon, you have to train – to put yourself under discipline. This requires making it habitual.

Habits

'A habit is a 3-step neurological process. First, there's a cue, something that tells your brain to go into automatic mode. Then there's a routine. And finally, a reward, which helps your brain learn to crave the behaviour.'

Duhigg

Changing a habit can be a bit like attempting to fill in the Grand Canyon to stop the flow of the Colorado River. Instead, it is easier to start at the source and divert it down a different initial path. One of the simplest ways is to use something that you already do as a cue.

My suggestion is getting up when the alarm clock goes off. Set that as a trigger for a simple, enjoyable and possibly energising morning routine to be intentional. For example, mine looks like this.

> When the alarm goes at 6:45:
> I will get up and make a cup of tea, and then
> I will contemplate the Bible passages for the day, and then
> I will get up and go to my desk, and then
> I will plan the day considering my quarterly and weekly goals, and then
> I will journal what I am grateful for, and then
> I will pray for God's help through the day, and then
> I will shower and get breakfast…

Obviously, your plan will be different to this, but notice how it contains an element of purpose, discipline and mindfulness.

You might choose to use some kind of quiet practice where I contemplate the Bible. You may insert your own morning exercise or stretching routine instead of making a cup of tea. The key point here is to *avoid mindlessness*, as that will enable the opposite.

Practice

'If people knew how hard I worked to get my mastery, it would not seem so wonderful at all.'

Michelangelo Buonarroti

We live in a talent-dominated culture, one where we have been led to believe that some fortunate few souls have been gifted by the gods with powers and abilities that somehow transcend those of us who are less blessed. We have all been given unique gifts, but these are not so much 'talents' as built-in areas of interest. It is left up to us to make the effort to spark them into life and fan the flames.

Our music and sporting arenas are filled with people labelled as 'talented' – those who are slated as overnight successes. However, deep down we know this not to be true. Find an interview with any top-flight sportsman or musician and notice that they routinely deny they have any talent, instead pointing to hours of practice. Talent is not, I believe, an in-built ability, more an in-built enthusiasm, drive and desire to do something of personal meaning. That interest may be sparked into life by a chance meeting or experience, which in turn generates an inner drive to practice.

Maria Montessori, the Italian educator, designed activities for children that were aimed at building specific skills, and they were allowed to repeat them for as long as they wanted. At the Montessori nursery that my children went to, this included activities such as cutting paper, pouring water, drawing in sandboxes and so on – just the kind of things that drive the parent of a pre-schooler nuts. Montessori's premise was that this was something in which the child felt they needed to develop skills, and interrupting them was frequently the cause of toddler tantrums.

Of course, as we grow up, we start practising more useful things – like maths.

Loving long division

There was a time when I struggled with maths and my lovely granny – a former teacher – made me a practice book, showed me how to do long division until I understood the process, then patiently gave me sums to do. I still remember sitting at the kitchen table, repeatedly begging 'give me two really long numbers, granny'.

Even now, I will reach for a pencil and a bit of paper when I need to do some long division, just because I find it fun. You could say I have a talent for it. However, the practice was not fun when I could not get it to 'come out', and I had to push through resistance until I could do it repeatedly, as and when needed.

A few years ago, thanks to Malcolm Gladwell, we all learned about the 10,000 hours rule: to achieve mastery in a task, we need 10,000 hours on task. Digging into this in more detail, it turned out that the number came from a detailed study of world-class violinists, was found to be different for differing skills, and potentially flawed – as the numbers were all self-reported rather than being measured.

The moral of this story is: let go of there being a magic number – the secret is all in the practice. For example, find a video of Chinese Olympic divers training: you will see how the dives are broken down into constituent parts and rehearsed again and again, day after day, until they can be reliably and accurately repeated. Once the elements are learned and in the so-called 'muscle memory', they are reassembled into a dive. It is hard, physical work on the surface, and watching the faces of the divers tells us of mental work that is going on too. We cannot see their inner thoughts, but they look bored, anxious and, at times, puzzled (will it be worth all this in the end?).

Talent is created through practice – boring, difficult, monotonous and possibly even painful repetition. What a highly skilled musician such as Ed Sheeran really has is the ability to endure that kind of mental and physical pain, doing enough to be able to perform in a way that appears fun and effortless. However, we must not be confused into thinking that if it is not fun, we are never going to get there. That is another lie our culture tells us: that when it starts to get a little too hard, we are not going to be successful and would be better off giving up.

Nevertheless, what has this got to do with resilience? By working out what enables us to build our resilience, we can break it down into component parts to be learned, and practise until they become a part of us. Much like Ed Sheeran's guitar playing, Shaiku Kane-Mason's cello playing, or Mo Farah's marathon running. The only difference is that when they put their 'skills' to the test, it is usually up to them; while for us, it probably will not be. But that is even more reason to push through the pain – to learn skills and turn them into talents.

'*Training* is the development of the mind or character or both, or some faculty, at some length, by exercise, as a soldier is trained or drilled. *Discipline* is essentially the same as *training, but more severe*' (*Century Dictionary*; emphasis added). Is it the severity aspect that makes discipline distasteful in our modern world? We only tend to start applying this kind of focused effort when we have a significant target to achieve, whether that might be hitting a repeated daily level of achievement, or doing the reading necessary to get through our next promotion exams.

Discipline needs to feature more largely in our lives. In areas such as:

- how we use our time (especially mornings and evenings)
- how we prepare for each day
- getting enough sleep
- eating enough of the right things (and not too much of the bad stuff), and so on.

Building our resilience for the future requires this kind of discipline. By the end of this book, you will probably have a number of things to put into a resilience development plan. While discipline may be an old-fashioned term in today's culture, its benefits are as applicable to us and our resilience as they were when St Paul wrote:

> Every athlete exercises self-control in all things. They do it to receive a perishable wreath, but we an imperishable. So I do not run aimlessly; I do not box as one beating the air. But I discipline my body and keep it under control (lest after preaching to others I myself should be disqualified). (Paul's first letter to the Corinthians, Chapter 9, v 25-27vv)

Waiting until you are in a chaotic situation is not the best time to realise that it would have been helpful to have avoided the cakes in the office for the last three months, or just simply had enough sleep the night before. Daily discipline = resilience reinforcement.

Next steps

1. In which areas of your life are you most, and least, disciplined? What can you learn from one in order to improve the other?
2. What regular daily, disciplined action can you take that will build your resilience, based on what we have considered so far?

14. Planning

'When you plan each day in advance, you find it much easier to get going and to keep going... you feel more powerful and competent. You eventually become *unstoppable*.'

Brian Tracy

Obviously, the secret to success is starting out on the right foot. As Chris Chesney, Global Practice Leader for Execution at Franklin Covey, writes in *The 4 Disciplines of Execution* (2012), it is important to have the right number of goals to be working on: for example, Franklin Covey found that where teams had more than 11 significant goals, they achieved none of them.

Apart from the sheer overhead of running that number of projects, the issue is most likely and primarily to do with switching (which we will cover when we look at effectiveness, in Chapter 12). The result of achieving none of our major goals is that we end each day feeling that we have worked hard but achieved nothing, which depletes our morale, drive and possibly self-esteem – especially if it continues over an extended time, as it erodes our resilience.

A never-ending merry-go-round

As someone owning and running my own business, there is always something to be done. If I am not running a workshop, then I am likely to be designing a new one, talking to a customer, doing the accounts, payroll or VAT return. It's a never-ending merry-go-round – and that is before an endless stream of questions and ideas. For a long time I felt that I had not achieved anything on most days.

One day over a family supper, Emily asked about my day.

'Meh, rubbish.'
'But why? At lunch you said that you'd had three useful phone calls, started designing a workshop, designed and ordered some workbooks, which sounds like a lot to me.'
'Ah yes, but there's so much to do, and I didn't get any of it done.'

'Well, what did you plan? Didn't you have any outcomes for those things?' (She is studying psychology, what can I say!)

As it turned out, there were so many significant things on my list that I was basically spinning on the spot. If I was doing the accounts, I felt bad because I was not doing any marketing, and if I was doing marketing, I felt bad because I was not writing and so on.

The problem was that I did not have any outcomes mapped. My resilience to anything going wrong in the business was low, because I was constantly chasing my tail. When it did (and there is always something!), then pretty much everything was dropped to deal with it, and I felt bad all over again.

It was time to get my house in order. More correctly, to get my *outcomes* in order.

It is obvious that we should have some kind of plan for our days. What we will do, where, when and with whom. If you want an easier life, consider creating a 'foundation plan' for each day of the week containing all the things that you routinely have to do. The discipline will set you free, and give you confidence.

With so much on our plates, it is so tempting to dive straight into action rather than taking a few minutes to scan the horizon and consider the bigger picture.

Problem clarity

First, we need to be sure that we have absolute clarity on the problem that we are trying to solve. These questions should facilitate that. If you can't answer them, then there is still more work to be done! I came up with the TIP model to help:

- **Truth** – what is the real situation, not just the one you are telling yourself?
- **Impact** – what impact is the situation having on you or someone else, or both?
- **Prefer** – what would you (or they) rather have happen (or be)?

Using 'personal wellbeing' as an example, our answers might be:

- **T** – Working excessive hours, not making time to rest, exercise, get fresh air or enough sleep.

- **I** – Constantly running on empty, tired and grumpy – which is tough for my family.
- **P** – Feeling on top of things, able to ride the bumps of everyday life.

The outcome map

Once you have clarity on the problem that you are trying to solve, you are well placed to use an outcome-based approach to explore the other factors that will help you to be more successful. Figure 7 (on the next page) presents an example template.

Working this through with a recent participant on the FLAME programme (a one-to-one development model for middle and senior managers, which we will cover in Chapter 24), we reduced the original map to a version that was more immediately applicable to their context. The aim was twofold: to create clarity of direction, as well as a compelling vision for action – ensuring that we are seeing the bigger picture.

What do you actually want?

The first branch is: 'What do you want?' This seems blindingly obvious, I know. While clarifying the problem using TIP initiates our thinking, there are some additional things to consider.

Often, what we say we want is phrased negatively: 'I want to stop X' or 'I want less Y'. It is critical that an outcome or goal statement is towards-motivated and framed positively. It needs to avoid 'want', 'should', 'could' or 'ought', as these words point in the direction of something we *do not* want!

Our brains do not differentiate between real and imagined, positive or negative – they are all treated equally, so we need to focus on what we actually want. 'You can't do a don't', as my friend Paul puts it. Maybe you will need to ask yourself questions along the lines of 'If I didn't have that problem, what would happen?' in order to shift your thinking. Sticking with the wellbeing example and building on the earlier thoughts, this might be: 'I want to prioritise taking care of myself while still keeping others safe.'

Pausing to thoroughly evaluate the real objective overcomes any tendencies we may have to jump too swiftly from 'why' to 'what' and 'how'. Just try to live with the tension for now. It will be resolved when the map is completed!

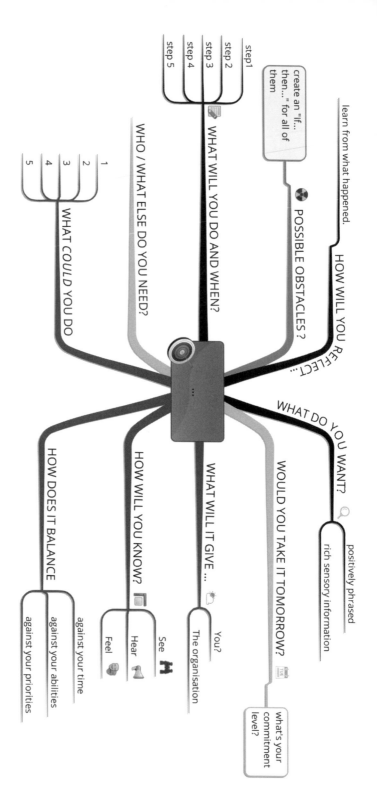

Figure 7: An outcome-based approach

What will it give you?

The next branch is about evaluating the benefits of achieving the task. It is worth considering at least three viewpoints, which would include you and your organisation. The third could be an offender, an external agency, and/or the victim of a crime. Doing this triangulation may highlight some undesirable consequences for one of the parties, meaning that you will have to decide if the overall outcome is acceptable.

Completing this branch not only enriches our understanding of the task, but also builds our motivation towards achieving it. Continuing our example, this might be:

> I will feel a greater sense of balance in my life, that I am able to ride the wrinkles of everyday work and life. As a result, I'll be able to deliver a better service to the public, represent my service better, and my family and friends will get the best of me.

What will the evidence be?

Research done on goal setting and mental contrasting by Gollwitzer et al. (2011) shows that by considering what it will be like when a goal is completed, we are more likely to achieve it than if we just got on with it. So for this branch we are thinking about the three main senses.

The description of our goal needs to be 'technisense' – rich in sensory information – to make it as real as possible. Everything becomes real to our brain if we make it vivid enough. The key is to cover the three main senses: visual, auditory and kinaesthetic. It helps to imagine the task as already completed by asking ourselves: 'What will it be like when…?' Moreover, it will be evidence that *you are making progress* – this helps when you hit one of those inevitable obstacles which we shall consider shortly. It also helps you track your progress easily.

Think about this from both an internal and external perspective:

- What might you hear in your inner voice?
- What words would you hear from another person?
- What might you see yourself and others doing?

Make sure that you cover all of these perceptual positions, as we all have a preference for which of these senses we use. Considering all of them provides a richer and more motivating representation.

In our example:

- **Auditory**: 'I'll be telling myself that I'm fitter. I'll hear my family saying I'm more fun to be around.'
- **Visual**: 'I'll see myself reacting to events in a more measured way. I'll see the team calmer.'
- **Kinaesthetic**: 'I'll feel rested, calmer and healthier.'

Options and actions

Now we can think about the 'how'. These next two branches need little explanation. When coming up with options, you need a minimum of four. If you are struggling to do so, then you can have some fun playing a 'What if?' mind game of the form:

- What would a famous person (e.g. Arianna Huffington) do?
- What would my favourite film/play/book character do?
- What would be a radical approach?
- What would be counter-intuitive?
- What would be the 'fool's view' – the negative opposite to the outcome I want?

What you are going to do and when is now more of a simple scheduling task, but it still needs detail in the temporal elements. Defining a completion milestone as 'the end of Wednesday 14th', is too open to interpretation – imagine if the responsible person is on a late shift that day. When they think the task has to be completed, and when you do, could be totally different!

Preparing for obstacles

We must consider the possible obstacles that might emerge as we progress. Gollwitzer et al.'s (2011) research also showed that by using 'mental contrasting' (comparing the expected outcome with what might go wrong along the way), the likelihood of success is increased still further.

As before, you may need to adopt multiple perceptual positions to come up with a reasonable set. Use the same actors as you did earlier, including the ones who might be adversely impacted by your success. Once you have identified potential obstacles and workarounds for each, it may be necessary to refine or supplement the timescales from the previous step.

Reflection

Behind every event in our lives lies a learning opportunity: it just depends whether you choose to see it as such. Simply identify how and when you will reflect on what happens – and remember to include multiple check-ins during a longer task.

Application

Taking an outcome-centred approach such as this orients us towards a solution-focused way of thinking: a core feature of resilience. It has proved to be useful to all aspects of life, whether thinking alone or in a group context. Here are three potential applications.

Visioning

Where a task requires a team-based approach, one of the most significant challenges is to get everyone to see the same vision and buy into what needs to be done. Building a map like this together with the team will achieve both of these.

Better still, it will enable you to delegate with confidence and thus empower your staff. Often, when everyone has been part of creating the outcome, you can let them decide the most appropriate way to act (within the scope of your standard operating procedures, of course). This was one of the things that Commander L. David Marquet (2012) uncovered through captaining the *USS Olympia*.

Decisions

I shared this model in a workshop as one of the ways of building a high-performing team. One delegate told me how she had gone to a decision-making meeting, expecting it to take at least two hours; however, by using the map above and completing it together with the group at the start of the meeting, they reached a conclusion within 30 minutes. Even better, there was a high level of engagement and agreement on the conclusion.

Meetings

We all know the best way to run effective meetings: agendas set in advance, material circulated in good time, papers read in advance, etc. But we do not always do that work upfront, for any number of reasons. While there is no real alternative to good preparation, using the following approach can go some way to alleviating that.

Just spend the first few minutes of the meeting completing one of these maps together: you may be pleasantly surprised by what happens. One team I work with found that this method shortened making a tough decision from an expected 90 minutes to little more than 30 minutes. It can also build engagement.

When you consider each of these aspects for building your resilience, and preparing for a major task, goal or outcome, it will help you (and possibly your team) to be clearer about what you are trying to achieve. Moreover, it could save you time and empower them to action. Finally, it will prove invaluable in a complex, unplanned event – so it is part of building your resilience for the future.

Outcome-focused thinking

Thinking in terms of outcomes is critical if we are to be more resilient, because by really getting to the heart of a goal or objective, evaluating the options, considering the potential obstacles and planning for them, we are better equipped to deal with challenges, as well as being more motivated to keep going when things get tough.

By using this as part of your day-to-day work, when it is required in a crisis situation the thinking process will have become automatic.

How should you use this approach? Of course, the best way is with paper and pencil.

Next steps

1. Create an outcome map for each of your annual or quarterly goals, preferably with the team involved in delivering them.
2. Try using the outcome map to create the agenda for a meeting at the outset.
3. Try using this map to design an event, and learn from what happens.
4. When you reach the end of this book, use this to plan your own approach to some of the key activities you are going to undertake to build your own resilience.

15. Distractions

'Distractions are everywhere. And with the always-on technologies of today, they take a heavy toll on productivity.'

David Rock

Where do our distractions come from? My guess is that 80 per cent are from within us. Some of those are due to not using our PETs effectively: going back to the example in Chapter 12, I am more likely be distracted at 2 pm, when my energy level is low and I have lower willpower.

The reason that there are tempting sweeties at the checkout in the supermarket is that willpower is a limited resource. Having spent a lot of willpower deciding not to buy that great deal on a bottle of fizz, or resisting luscious chocolate puddings, it is depleted by the time you load up at the checkout, and so you think 'Chocolate? Absolutely! I'm a bit peckish after all that shopping...'

So, where are you wasting yours? There is something to do with time of day that influences how easily distracted we can be – and there is also something about our personalities (which we looked at in Chapters 8 and 9, on drivers and temperament). Let's now consider how these give us inner 'time-pirates' to battle against in our quest for effectiveness.

Drivers

As we saw in Part 2, drivers are an in-built part of us of which we are often unaware and cause us to behave in certain ways, especially when under pressure. Here we are considering how those drivers show up.

Strength

The strength driver can look like time-pirates who will defend the ship of achievement single-handedly. The trouble is that no one else grows when we do this, and we can end up burned out and resentful.

One answer could be to find something small that you can ask for help with, and create plans which include the 'me time' that you know you need. You will end up developing your own ability to get the best out of others, as well as reducing your own risk of burnout.

Try this self-talk: 'It is OK to show my emotions. To be real and let people know what's going on. I'm going to use that inner strength to recognise and ask for help when I need it.'

Perfectionism

With a perfectionism driver you feel the need for everything to be just right (a bit like those of us with a Guardian temperament). You may have to rework your list of priorities and plans endlessly – almost as if that is the end in itself. But a plan is like scaffolding, and just there to support the real work. Beat this time-pirate by doing what works and doing it now, accepting that it is more important to finish on time than to be as perfect as you might want it to be.

Self-talk: 'Good enough is good enough, it's more important to finish on time.'

Helpfulness

This sneaky time-pirate will have you doing almost anything for almost anyone else before yourself. So beat it into submission by just getting started and letting your actions speak for you, rather than constantly and solely focusing on others.

Self-talk: 'I'm going to say what I think, get on with doing it, and take care of myself every day. Put myself first for a change.'

Persistence

Constantly trying hard creates time-pirates who never know when to stop – perhaps taking on too much simultaneously. Conquer them by doing one thing at a time and planning to follow through with a clear vision of the completed state.

Self-talk: 'This is what I need to get done. Keep the main thing in focus.'

Busyness

The busyness driver sees us not preparing because there is never enough time, as well as being regularly late (again, because we never leave enough time) – so we find planning difficult. We feel that there is no time to waste, and just want to get on with everything. We find it hard to judge how long things take, and the energy required.

A counter attack against this thief of the sea of time is to take small steps, breaking tasks up into bite-sized activities.

Self-talk: 'It is OK to start early and take my time. I'm going to enjoy being on time.'

Temperament

As we saw in Part 2, temperament is that in-built part of you, who you are at your core. These are clues to your inner saboteurs too. With awareness of how your temperament might contribute to these particular time-pirates, you can start working out how to play to its strengths, rather than just crossing swords.

Guardian time-pirates

With a Guardian temperament, you like things to be orderly. With a natural talent for ensuring that the right things are in the right place at the right time, you find building a task list easy. However, simultaneously, with your need for things to be 'done correctly', it may take you a long time to get your task list or big picture plan together.

You may feel the need to have your boss make sure you are doing what is expected: your naturally cautious and 'Eeyore nature', expecting things to go wrong in the future, may be more of a saboteur to you rather than the protector it usually is.

To win the battle with Guardian-led time-pirates, try giving yourself permission to accept things for how they are, and use your drive for organisation to plan forward rather than dwelling backward. More importantly, allow yourself to proceed in hope, rather than having to wait for approval while expecting the worst.

Idealist time-pirates

If you have an Idealist temperament, your intuitive nature may lead you to disregard the need for a list, big picture plan or even prioritisation, preferring instead to trust your naturally strong gut instinct. Your eagerness to make sure that you take people with you harmoniously, empower and grow them, may make that more of a challenge too. With such a strong desire to be helpful to others, you may be led more by their demands than those of the organisation, giving you an inner tension that can be hard to resolve.

Idealist time-pirates can be conquered by not ignoring what your gut tells you, but tempering it by prioritising your task list. Use that to create a more detailed list of things to do (think about it in terms of laying bricks to build a house, rather than building the whole thing). Imagining yourself at some future moment in time and looking back to the present day can help, as you see the benefits of a different approach and, in turn, its impact on others.

Rational time-pirates

If you have a Rational temperament, whatever you do needs to make logical sense to you. So you may spend a lot of time making sure that your list is aligned with the rest of itself, as well as your mission – at the expense of making real progress!

Your need for precision and to show how ingenious you are can derail you into spending a lot of time trying to figure out the optimal method to achieve something, rather than starting it. Then there is technology: your love for it can lead you down similar diversions – 'I wonder which app is best for this?', or 'How could this system be better?'

Rational temperament-driven time-pirates can be overcome by seeking an external viewpoint, as well as entertaining the possibility that an imprecise plan might be of greater value than one that is highly detailed and has taken ages to construct. Time-boxing – working within a pre-defined limited window of time – can help you avoid the diversions that you would normally take.

Artisan time-pirates

If, like me, you have an Artisan temperament, you will not want any kind of list or plan, as it feels as if it is tying you down excessively and blocking your need for variety. You are a natural in a crisis, and feel a need to act on impulse. Sadly, this can make you the best procrastinator in the room – waiting until the last minute just makes it all so much more exciting, doesn't it! Not for everyone else, though.

You are the eternal optimist about the future, knowing that things will turn out OK in the end. Just try imagining how much easier it could be to start early, to give you more time for fun later.

Artisan time-pirates seek swashbuckling action on the high seas, so with a desire for variety, try simply planning in smaller units of time (20 minutes, perhaps), with regular breaks in-between (but do be aware of the impact of task switching!). Just remember to take all your estimates and double them, to keep these pesky pirates at bay.

External distractions

Meetings

We have looked at the 80 per cent of internal distractions. What about the remaining 20 per cent – the external ones? What can we do about those? You may say you have to be available 100 per cent of the time for your boss or your team, but that is a judgement call – which is more important to you?

Sometimes it is about setting expectations. Imagine that you have a meeting scheduled for one of your key annual targets, which involves several of your external agencies to move it forward. You get a message from the personal assistant to your boss's boss asking you to attend a meeting at the same time. Attending that and delaying your own meeting will push back your project by four weeks.

Knowing your priorities and interdependencies is critical here. Having a clear outcome and knowing what you want from that meeting enables you to respond to the personal assistant and ask the question: 'Project X will be delayed by at least four weeks if I come to your meeting. What would you rather have me do?'

People

Today, many of us work in open-plan offices. The most common form of interruption here is often referred to as a 'drive by' or 'doorstepping'.

Somebody pauses at your desk, knocks on it (or the door, if you're lucky enough to have one of those). The most common form of this is: 'Have you got a minute?' How long do these actually take? Depending on the person, about 30 minutes. Assuming you can see that it is not a critical issue, a good answer is: 'Yes, you can have a minute now, or you can have 30 minutes at 3.30 pm.' Often when you get to 3.30 pm, the thing that they were going to ask you has either gone away, or someone else has helped them – and maybe they will not have to ask you next time.

Stopping doorstepping

The office I worked in 15 years ago provided us with a set of green ear defenders. Ostensibly to keep things quiet, but they also provided a visual cue that you were not to be interrupted. You might have a phone headset, which will do just as well – generally we think someone with one of these on is in a teleconference. A pair of earbuds does not work quite as well, as we all know that while they might be on the phone, they are more likely to be listening to music. There are lower-tech solutions too – such as a red sticky note posted on the corner of your screen, the back of your chair or the divider between you and the next desk to indicate 'Do not disturb'.

Another problem with cube farms is that someone more than 10 metres away from us is more likely to send an electronic message than come over to our desk.

While that is useful when they glance across and see us with our headset on – and conclude that we are in a teleconference – it can rob us of some interpersonal contact that would improve our resilience.

Personal digital assistants

Back in the early 1990s, the newest must-have device was a personal digital assistant (PDA). For the first time ever, you could synchronise your computer calendar and address book with a pocket-sized bit of electronics, which meant that you could check where you were meant to be, and look up contacts' phone numbers at any time. It did not do email, but it did have a nifty touchscreen area which you could 'write' on with a stylus – and once you had learned the modified version of the alphabet, you could take notes or create new diary entries. All very exciting.

It did not take companies such as Apple and BlackBerry very long to realise that a phone could be integrated with this mobile diary thing, and so the smartphone was born. If you remember back that far, the iPhone originally had room for 20 app icons on the front screen. The latest iPhone has 32. It is said that Steve Jobs would not allow his children to have an iPad when it first launched, because he foresaw that it would be used by developers to entrap users within their environments and lead to great swathes of people glued to these PDAs – now Personal Distraction Agents.

Try going to the notification screen on your phone: scroll through and see how many pages you have. Do you realise that you have given permission to most of them to disturb you at practically any time? Of course, that includes useful things such as train and flight times, but also less useful prompts such as social media updates.

We have created a tool to distract ourselves, and we take it practically everywhere. Not really an assistant anymore, is it?

The amount of time we spend within the digital world is scary, and getting worse. Designer and developer Kevin Holesh was interested in exactly how much, so he built *Moment* – an app to help us understand how addicted we are to these lightweight time thieves. Recent research by Kliener Perkins Caufield Byers (KPCB) showed that in 2017 we each spent 5.9 hours a day using digital media. Of that, 3.3 hours were accessed via a mobile device – that is up from under an hour in 2011. (Data from the *Moment* app is on a par with this, in case you doubt it.)

Read Adam Alter's *Irresistible* for a more in-depth exploration of the situation, but it is clear that we are enslaved to these digital devices. You only have to go out of reach of Wi-Fi and/or 4G to find out how regularly you are 'just checking'. That may be the biggest issue – not just the lost (wasted, even) time – but the fact that we are constantly distracted. Even as I have been writing this, looking up the references, I have been distracted into reading at least three articles on *Lifehacker* about other things that, seconds ago, were more interesting. This kind of 'just checking' has a significant cognitive overload: research shows that the habit of task switching costs from 15 to 25 minutes of lost concentration because of 'attention residue' (Leroy, 2009).

Imagine you are writing a report: it isn't very interesting. So you click to your email inbox, where you see a long list of headlines and opening paragraphs. Within it, there is one message that catches your eye – so you open it, read it, don't take any action and then switch back to the report that you were working on before. For at least the next 15 minutes, you will be thinking at some level about the email you just read. You make some progress on your report, but you will not be doing the deep work necessary to have a significant impact until you have been focusing for 15 minutes.

Now, imagine if you just check only four times an hour. Your deep work effectiveness in that hour is zero. According to Holesh, from the data collected via his app *Moment* (on December 2018) shows that the average *Moment* user picks their phone up 55 times a day, spending 3 hours and 57 minutes on it. If each of those 'just checks' has an attention residue of 15 minutes, that equates to over 13 hours of shallow work each day.

Never mind the loss of the 3 hours, it is a miracle that we get anything done at all. In *Deep Work*, Cal Newport shows us that the people who are most likely to be successful in the future are those who can focus on significant packages of work for *extended periods*.

So, what can you do? Well, you can start turning off some of those notifications on your phone – and your computer.

Email

How do you have your messages sorted? The default is by date, because we believe that the most important messages are the most recent ones; but that just sets us up with a Pavlovian response to email, and can be a massive distraction. If you change the default to sort by person, it is much easier to find what you are looking for before closing email altogether.

Another thing is CC'd messages. Why do we CC someone? Often, just to cover ourselves! And what about 'Reply All'? How much fun is it to watch the chain grow with messages that say 'Please can you take me off this list?', or better still 'Please don't reply all'!

Coping with the CC's

Ten years ago, as a worldwide development manager at Hewlett-Packard, I was getting between 80 and 100 emails a day. It was unbearable. The main thing I needed to do each day was to find the messages from the people that were most important.

In MS Outlook you can change settings to display messages in varying colour and font sizes by sender. So I set up messages from my boss to appear in 20pt red text, and CC'd messages in 8pt grey text. As a result, it was really easy to see the messages that I needed to deal with first. You might try something similar.

Instead of this randomness, agree some email etiquette with your team. For example: messages that require action from someone must have them on the To line, and others who might need to know on the CC line. Then you can set up a rule to siphon off CC'd messages to a separate folder to read when you get time (if at all). I did this with my team at Hewlett-Packard, and it made a big difference.

However, there is a health warning with this. A police officer I was talking to recently, complained vociferously about a colleague who had an auto-responder to CC'd messages which said something like: 'I treat CC'd messages as low priority, so if it's important please resend TO me.' It is all about setting expectations.

The biggest problem by far is the volume of email that we *send*. Unless you have subscribed to lots of email news, the volume of what you send directly correlates with the volume you get. There is an obvious win-win when you get up and talk to someone, instead of just sending them an email. Try not always jumping in to answer every question – there are always lots of other people who can do that, so let them. You don't have to use every email to demonstrate your advanced knowledge or educate people.

No doubt you have your laptop set up to open email automatically. Why is that? By routinely checking email as the first activity in your day, you hand over your agenda, plans and aspirations to whomever has sent you a message. Why would you be doing email in your PETs anyway? Probably because that is what you think is expected – but have you actually checked that out?

Lots of us have accepted the default setup where a pop-up appears to alert you that new email has arrived. This gives you yet another opportunity to be distracted by 'just checking'. It can – and probably should be – turned off when you don't need to be informed of every new message.

I can hear your screams even now. 'But people will complain if I don't respond to their email in 10 seconds!' The Boston Consulting Group did an experiment with one of its teams, forbidding team members from doing any email for one day a week in rotation. There was a lot of resistance, as you can imagine. The teams' customer reported that they had made more progress than in a typical week, and that they had not noticed anything different.

Better email expectations

I heard recently of a chief constable who banned the use of email before 12 pm – saying that if people really wanted one another's attention or help, they should use the phone instead. Seems radical, doesn't it? It is not so much of a challenge to change this kind of thing, because it is really only about setting expectations.

The biggest problem with email is that we are almost addicted to it. We need to set more realistic expectations. Perhaps not opening email until you have done at least an hour on your most important goal during your PETs. (After all, why would you open email during a time when you know that you are at your peak effectiveness?)

Are you up for changing the culture of email in this way? I really hope so, because we have handed over our lives to the inbox and it is time to take it back. The good news is you are in a strong position to influence this. The bad news? You will have to set the example. Choose to start actively setting and managing people's expectations of when you are (and are not) going to be available.

Use these, and reflect

Having taken several different viewpoints of how we allow our personal time-pirates to steer our ship off course, you will have had some insights into what you might do differently to thwart them.

Awareness of how these affect us when we are calm helps us to see how they exert greater influence when we become stressed; so working with them in mind will increase your resilience for those times when things become more pressured. When you find yourself in a challenging situation, take the opportunity to reflect on small changes that you could make to improve things, or even just understand what is going on for you – which will increase your sense of control.

It is worth reiterating the need for regular reflection too – and an experimental nature – i.e. try something, see what works and do more of that. This is not going to be an overnight transformation, but increased awareness will enable you to make multiple, small corrections to your course which have a larger impact over time.

Next steps

1. If you have not done so already, find out your drivers and temperament.
2. Are you more influenced by the time-pirates resulting from your drivers or from your temperament? Plan how you are going to conquer them.
3. When could you switch off email? Who do you have to change (or validate) your assumptions regarding responding to email or instant messages? With whom do you need to create some email etiquette?

16. Prioritisation

'The man who hunts two rabbits catches neither.'

Chinese proverb

With our scope of work continuing to soar as resources seem to sink, it is far too easy to just pick the next thing to work on from the top of our inbox, instead of taking the time to prioritise properly. If you ever get to the end of your day feeling that you have not actually achieved anything of value, the chances are you did not get the priorities right – if, indeed, you prioritised at all! We know this but still struggle to do anything different, for all the reasons mentioned under 'Distractions' (Chapter 15).

Wouldn't it be better if there were a quick way to pause, take stock and set off in a purposeful direction instead?

Why is prioritisation so difficult?

For anything other than a simple shopping list, there are multiple dimensions to consider. The first of those is how you use your head – or put better, how your brain acts. Functional Magnetic Resonance Imaging (fMRI) shows that the prefrontal cortex of the human brain is used for so-called 'executive functions' such as focusing, thinking and evaluation (as well as helping us task-switch and tune out distractions).

Two things are important for us to know about the prefrontal cortex. First, it has a small capacity (just like having a low amount of storage for pictures on your phone); second, it consumes a lot of energy as it does its work. Trying to think of what to do *and* what order to do it in has a large cognitive load, and therefore is harder to do, the longer the list. If your energy level is already low (because you have not eaten, for example), just trying to do this can lead you to feel weak, liable to distraction and even nauseous. It is like driving on the opposite side of the road when you first roll off the ferry abroad – you can't even have the radio on because you need to concentrate so much.

Often we take the easy way out with prioritising, by just choosing one item, getting it done and so on. The problem is that this can lead us to being too gut-driven in our choices, and thus our actions.

An obvious initial step is to get the list recorded. With research showing that we are more likely to retain information that we write rather than type, the best way is to do it on paper, with a pen. Then we need to apply a repeatable process. There are several such processes, from simple (e.g. MoSCoW Rules – Must, Should, Could and Won't – from agile software development techniques) to complex (e.g. the CARVER matrix). Here is one that I have created that sits between those two.

The ROME matrix

R stands for Risk – how much risk is there to yourself or others if this is not done?

O stands for Others – how important is this to others, e.g. senior staff, the person involved?

M stands for Me – how important is this to me personally?

E stands for Emotion – how strong is my gut reaction?

The method is to consider each perspective in turn and score all tasks against one another from 1–5 (where 1 is lowest and 5 is highest), then add the scores together. The highest total score wins the priority race.

Table 3 shows how this might play out for a fictitious task list for a police officer.

Activity	ROME rating				
	R	**O**	**M**	**E**	**Total**
Serious welfare case	4	5	4	4	17
Child abuse disclosure	5	5	4	5	19
Vulnerable adult abuse disclosure	5	5	4	4	18
Personal wellbeing activity	3	2	5	4	14
Burglary investigation	3	4	3	3	13
Personal development	1	2	5	4	12
Grievous bodily harm (GBH) investigation	4	5	4	4	17
One-to-ones with staff	2	4	4	2	12
New crime allocation process	1	5	1	1	8

Table 3: The ROME matrix

In this example, using the ROME matrix to prioritise the day will result in one of the disclosures rising to the top of the list, closely followed by the other, and the welfare and GBH cases into third and fourth respectively. Notice that, with this approach, our personal development drops way down the list.

If you have a sense that one dimension is generally more important than another in your context, then you could apply a weighting factor. For example, if Risk of harm to someone is much more important than your Emotional gut reaction, you could multiply your risk score by a factor of 2. Try to keep it simple, though. Alternatively, if two scores are equal, or very close together, multiply the factors instead of adding them, as suggested by Larry Mallak.

This approach is good where you have multiple stakeholders and need to justify your decision; however, it could still be seen as a little subjective, so you may want to record your reasoning as well. You may score each of these example tasks differently to me, but my hope is that through the worked example, you can see how you might apply this tool in real life.

While prioritisation is not an exact science – and there could be arguments for and against any model – using a process such as ROME will help you avoid constantly working in the 'urgent box' by balancing speed and precision – which can only make the job (and life) easier. Of course, it would be even better if you externalise your thinking by doing the prioritisation as a team – thus bringing them into your map of the world and setting them up as leaders rather than followers.

As with many of these facets, making prioritisation part of your daily discipline, alongside using your PETs effectively and managing distractions, will enable you to use your time more effectively. This will help you feel more in control of what is going on, and build your resilience too.

Next steps

1. Take your to-do list and prioritise it using ROME now. Validate it by finding a colleague to explain your choices.
2. Drawing on the previous chapters, build an outcome map for the top three items on your prioritised list from step 1. Consider the distractions that you are prone to, and develop mitigation strategies for each.

17. Exercise

'[After taking up running training properly] what I found even more interesting were the changes that had begun to take place in my mind. I was calmer and less anxious. I could concentrate more easily and for longer periods. I felt more in control of my life. I was less easily rattled by unexpected frustrations. I had a sense of quiet power, and if at any time I felt this power slipping away I could call it back by going out running... something in running has a uniquely salutatory effect on the mind.'

(Fixx, 1979)

Exercise is one area of building resilience where you probably need to take expert advice as well as applying personal discipline. My aim here is to provide clarity on the benefits – the 'why' rather than the 'how' – which, after all, has an entire industry around it!

Imagine that you had bank accounts for your physical and emotional health. Exercise makes a credit to both of them, and is therefore worthy of greater attention. The UK NHS crisis would probably be smaller if we all took greater responsibility for our own health and gave it the priority it deserved.

Top-flight sports people such as marathon runners not only consider a periodic training plan with sufficient hard work (e.g. hill running), easier slow distance runs, and musculoskeletal training, but also consider the impact of rest, sleep, nutrition and hydration. The rest of us do not have such needs, we rightly argue, but as a result seem to abandon all of them instead of considering what our own version of each might be.

Taking responsibility means doing similar things to these elite athletes: watching exercise levels, and so on. It is your body and your responsibility. Improving your physical state is a precursor to getting in better emotional shape – and is a virtuous cycle.

To be physically healthier usually requires better habits. However, often we have set ourselves up for behaviours that undermine our exercise and fitness goals. For example, eating a biscuit with a morning coffee. If you routinely reach for the biscuit barrel as the kettle boils, you are probably eating anything from 6 to 10 biscuits a day. That is more than half a packet! Put all those biscuits or snacks on a plate and imagine eating them in one sitting: gross, eh?

As we have seen, the secret of any habit is to start so small that it is almost negligible effort to achieve. For example, a 5-minute daily walk can easily turn into 30 minutes in less than a month, especially if you go with someone else. Sleeping properly will give you a physical recharge, obviously, and exercise will help you sleep better too (as long as you do not exercise too close to bedtime).

In a nutshell, exercise to improve your fitness will give you an increased sense of wellbeing, a calming effect on your mind, and helps relieve stress as well as being useful for anxiety and depression.

There is so much to be gained from something so simple. Consider how our grandparents got around – they did not have anything like a gym membership (which possibly only makes you feel more guilty when you don't allow enough time for it!). There is really no need for Lycra or leotards; just get some good shoes, a waterproof jacket and walk, or a bike and ride – and stick at it. Commit to it with some friends for 30 days, and just see what happens. I have known lots of folk who applied this to running and were soon, to their (and it has to be said, my) surprise, hooked.

As always, consider taking appropriate medical advice before taking up any new exercise regime.

Next steps

1. Decide to commit to achieving the government's exercise target for the next month. What will you do, with whom and when, precisely? Where? Do you need medical advice before starting out?
2. Build an outcome map for this exercise goal. Keep it to yourself, or perhaps share it with one other person who can hold you accountable.

18. Mindfulness

> 'It's up to me to mindfully respond or mindlessly react to whatever life brings.'
>
> (Charles Hunt, 2016)

Mindfulness is the word *du jour*. Depending on what you read and the beliefs you ascribe to, it can be anything from taking a quiet walk or carving out some personal quiet time. For me that means having a time of prayer and Bible contemplation. You may have a daily yoga practice, workout or meditation. Each to their own.

The benefits of being more mindful are clear through neuroscience and research driven from a general concern about wellbeing and mental health. According to the American Psychological Association (2012), it has been shown that practising some type of mindfulness (whether by pausing for a few minutes to become more curiously aware of our internal and external sensations, without placing any judgement on them or the outcome), or by guided meditation, can have some of the following positive results:

- Reduced depressive symptoms
- Improved working memory capacity
- Improved ability to focus
- Decreased anxiety
- Reduced stress
- Increased ability to regulate emotions

Notice for a moment how many of these are aspects of what wellbeing programmes are trying to achieve. Maybe we should ditch them entirely and just have 15 minutes' quiet time at the start (and probably, the end) of every day, when we can just be.

One interesting piece of research carried out at the University of Michigan has found that a short walk in natural surroundings can have similar effects – even to the point of just looking at pictures of natural environments (although obviously not with the physical benefits!).

Be here now

Part of being mindful is about being fully present – 'in the moment'. There's a well-known saying that goes something like, 'Yesterday is history, tomorrow is a mystery, today is a gift of God, which is why we call it the present.' So what can we do to be more present in the here and now?

Climbing to mindfulness

Sian, a rock-climber, told me how, when climbing up a rock face, all thoughts of work and the challenges there completely disappeared from her mind, as all she could think about was where the next hand or foothold would be, and how to keep from falling off.

The elation at reaching the top safely didn't see a return of negative thoughts of workload, but rather a shift in perspective that she realised also came from her daily mindfulness practice.

Sadly, we spend our days mindlessly moving from one thing to the next. We grab a cup of coffee and barely even notice the taste, or the smile on the barista's face – unless either are particularly striking. We walk to work with it, never noticing that spring is coming and trees are blossoming. We fail to see the glory of the creation around us. We grab a sandwich for lunch and eat it at our desk in an effort to be 'more efficient'. We don't notice what that tastes like really, either.

The word *mindless* has its roots in the 14th century, meaning 'unmindful, heedless, negligent'. Old English had the word *myndleas*, meaning foolish or senseless. We have forgotten what it really means to *be* rather than *do* – to be human *beings* rather than human *doings*. We rush everywhere, leaving little or no room for the unexpected, and consequently become stressed when things do not go quite as we planned.

All of this busyness has become habitual. Surely we should be taking every opportunity available to pause?

Some people don't know *how* to stop

Bannatyne's health clubs in the UK run a session called 'Body Balance'. This is a mixture of Tai Chi, yoga and Pilates aimed at overall stretching

---

and conditioning. Our local club has two different versions – one 60 minutes, the other 45, as I recently discovered.

Attending the 60-minute class by accident, we reached the end of the session and the trainer announced that we would be moving into the 'relaxation track'. With that, more than 50 per cent of the class got up from their mats and left. For me, it was a great opportunity to take 15 minutes to just stop and be, for my pulse rate to drop back to its normal level again.

Talking to the trainer afterwards, it turned out that this was normal behaviour. 'Some people,' she said, 'just don't seem to know *how* to stop.'

In the same way that we have a perceptual preference, we probably have a mindfulness preference. As a result, for your mindfulness practice, make sure that you include all of the senses within it. There are plenty of apps you can use on your phone – try some and see which works best for you. You can even find ones which combine this idea with building and maintaining focus – 'Tide' being just one example.

Twenty minutes to calm

At a recent workshop, when I asked participants if anyone practised mindfulness, Daniel talked about how practising meditation had changed his life.

Having recognised that he was getting burned out by work, and preferring to not get a supply of pills from his GP, he decided to try meditation.

Starting with as little as 2 minutes each day, it grew to 20 minutes. As a result, he noticed improvements in several areas of his life: most notably that now, when the need arose, he could take 20 minutes out and quieten himself, lower his heart rate and be calmer.

Knowing he has this tool at his disposal means he can endure the challenges that his work brings, rather than responding to them as threats. Even as he described his experience, it was noticeable that the rest of the room seemed to catch the calm.

Along with getting enough sleep (which we shall come to shortly) and getting clear on your SPP (which we covered in Chapter 4), this is one of the most important aspects of building a resilient life. What are you waiting for?

Next steps

1. Which of the benefits of mindfulness would be most advantageous to you? What difference will it make? (Remember to consider using the three senses.)

2. When, where and how are you going to create mindfulness in your life? Who or what help do you need, and how will you get it?

19. Reflection

'Everything that happens to you is your teacher. The secret is to learn to sit at the feet of your own life and be taught by it. Everything that happens is either a blessing which is also a lesson or a lesson which is also a blessing.'

Berrien Berends

If you have ever undertaken any kind of coaching or Neuro Linguistic Programming (NLP) training, you will have been asked to keep a journal so that you can evidence your experience, and build a web of continuous improvement. In my NLP training it was mandatory to do so.

Many of us take some time out on New Year's Day to set some resolutions. Doing this requires that we consider where we would like our life to be different, and that takes some reflection. However, the emphasis is very much on the 'new me', rather than the old one. We probably spend more time every year considering where to go on holiday than what has been going on in our lives. Apart, that is, from the first few days of holiday, when we are exhausted from trying to get our desks cleared before we left.

Just make some wood shavings

I know that I am poor at spotting my own stress levels. Indeed, during the final few years at Hewlett-Packard, it was Sue, my ever-patient wife, who would turn to me and say: 'You need to take a day off and make some wood shavings' – meaning 'You're becoming unbearable because you're too stressed to think straight.'

I was just too busy (and too tired at the day's end) to pause and reflect. Until, that is, I was wiped out with a colossal migraine or 'flu', which I took as my body's message to stop.

Apart from helping to manage stress, regular reflective practice can help us become more realistic about how much time we really have available for work and non-work activities, as well as evaluating where we need to work on ourselves.

I still have the journal from my NLP training. The content and the way I used it changed over time, but reviewing it now I can see a clear pattern emerge – that I would start journalling when things were tough, and stop when they improved again.

Eventually, I learned the lesson that it does not have to take long, be attractive, erudite or detailed; just that taking even 2 minutes every day and asking these five 'magic questions' helps to keep a handle on what is actually going on:

- What did you intend to do today?
- How hard did you try?
- What went well?
- What could have gone better?
- What will you do differently tomorrow?

When I realise that I am stressed, it is a simple matter to look back over the past two or three weeks and notice patterns. When faced with a repeated situation, I have something to build from, rather than guessing or starting over.

Embed through reflection

These questions emerged through a conversation with my friend Peter, who's a former Royal Marine. We were seeking ways to really embed learning for a leadership development programme for a police force, and I was curious as to what he saw as being different between how police officers were training and the Royal Marines.

Apart from the repetition, it was the fact that after each exercise, the platoon would gather and each take turns to answer questions like this. Only then would they have coffee and so forth, before going out and repeating the exercise until they got it right.

The benefits of journalling

Reading about journalling through history, there are many examples of how people have done this. I particularly like Benjamin Franklin's daily practice of considering each morning: 'What good shall I do this day?' and each evening the matching 'What good did I do this day?' Other people keep a diary, but often those are more about documenting life than reflecting on it.

Some favour a more creative approach to journalling – using particular colours for particular aspects (although I found it hard to remember which was for what, and kept losing the pens!). Others find that drawing or doodling as part of their reflective practice helps: indeed, there is a body of research into the impact of creative arts such as mosaic-making and pottery on resilience, and it seems particularly useful in the post-processing of traumatic events. (Kelly, 2012)

Choose any version you want, but stick to it for at least 12 weeks. If you chop and change more often than that, you will not be able to see what really works.

Practising gratitude

Following the positive psychology approach, it seems useful to add some kind of gratitude practice to our reflection. In *Flourish* (2011), Martin Seligman recommends writing down at least three things that we are grateful for, as his research showed that 'people who habitually acknowledge and express gratitude see benefits in their health, sleep, and relationships, and they perform better'.

I would add that they have to be things that are really meaningful for you, not just 'a beautiful sunset' – unless of course it was absolutely stunning!

Active reflection

As our emotional response to an event depends on how we think about it, then changing that inexorably changes our emotional response. While this is possible to do in the moment, it is a lot easier to learn to do through active reflection practice.

The annual year-end reflection has some value, but it doesn't have to be tied to then. How about choosing dates which have some personal significance, such as an anniversary, your birthday, the day before going on holiday or, come to that, the day after returning – which could be even better, as we tend to be more objective when we are rested. Just avoid letting it be only when you have a 'significant' life event, such as a birth or death. Why wait for these?

So far, we have looked at post-event reflection. Another type of reflection is the 'time out' – an in-the-midst-of-chaos reflection when we stop what we are doing, take a few deep breaths and step back both physically and mentally to review progress, plans and search for blind spots.

This type of reflection needs to engage as much of your physiology as possible – so, again, it is best done on paper with a pencil or pen. I have recently taken to using a pencil because it feels as if I am being creative at the same time (and it is easier to draw with, should I feel that way inclined).

Next steps

1. Decide which form of journalling you are going to try – formal notebook, informal cards, doodling or drawing. Get the materials you need, and schedule a 5-minute daily reflective practice for the next 28 days.

2. Find a buddy to do it alongside you, someone to whom you can be accountable for doing the reflection times, and share what you notice.

20. Self-compassion

> 'Self-compassion entails being kinder and more supportive toward oneself and less harshly judgmental. It involves greater recognition of the shared human experience, understanding that all humans are imperfect and lead imperfect lives, and fewer feelings of being isolated by one's imperfection. It entails mindful awareness of personal suffering, and ruminating less about negative aspects of oneself or one's life experience.'
>
> (Neff et al., in press)

The importance of self-care

Dr Kristen Neff is one of the world's foremost experts in this area, having defined the construct, researched it and developed a programme to teach self-compassion skills for daily life.

One of her key observations is that people who have a pet, such as a dog, will take more care of it than they will of themselves. For example, if a vet says that you need to apply cream to your dog's paw every 3 hours, you will set alarms and get up through the night; but if our doctor prescribes us some cream for an ailment, we would never dream of getting up through the night to apply it to ourselves. (Neff et al., 2018)

It seems that in the world today we are increasingly expected to sacrifice ourselves to achieve success. Work harder, get up earlier, 'You should' – worse still, 'I should'. It is as if we are all rushing around, constantly self-flagellating!

Beating yourself up

As a boy I once watched a military parade on a religious festival. Rank after rank of green-uniformed men marched down the city's main streets while beating themselves over alternate shoulders with a short piece of chain. To be in that particular army, you obviously had to be willing to beat yourself up.

If we were actually lazy, then a bit of personal agitation would be necessary. But are we? How many hours a week do you spend doing literally nothing? More to the point, how many hours a week do you spend doing anything that is purely for yourself? Probably precious few, and even those can induce feelings of guilt.

We need a little more compassion for ourselves. We are not perfect, and neither shall we ever be, so we can stop being so hard on ourselves. We know that harshness in the gym or out running will cause us an injury eventually.

We attend to our physical health and things such as our dental hygiene every day, having been taught about their importance from early in life, but we have not been taught about emotional and mental hygiene. It is bizarre that we never attend to the psychological injuries that often arise, but regularly attend to those physical ones (such as dental cavities) that occur infrequently. When I've had really bad toothache, I've gone to the dentist as soon as they can see me, but when I feel 'low' I tend to keep quiet about it and get through the day, hoping that I'll feel better tomorrow.

In a recent TED talk, psychologist Dr Guy Winch (2014) said: 'Loneliness creates a deep psychological wound that distorts our perception, making us believe that those around us care less than they actually do.' While we all have our own 'brand' of loneliness – one person's 'lonely' is another's 'lovely' – it is up to us to prioritise our emotional health through paying attention to our emotional pain. It is essential that we must first believe that this is possible, as it is too easy to convince ourselves otherwise. Telling ourselves that we are not worth others' attention or time is the equivalent of damaging that already broken arm.

Know thyself

'You do you' says author Sarah Knight in her own unique and often sweary way in her book *You Do You*. The point is this: know yourself, your limitations and weirdness, and cut yourself some slack. Rumination is one of our most unhelpful mental bad-health practices. Digging into negative thoughts and circling round can cause us significant impact.

To break the cycle, find a short, two-minute distraction and start countering this particular type of self-sabotage. Changing how you respond inside your head to what you see as failure, and battling to build your self-esteem by challenging this type of negative thinking, will build your emotional resilience. Cutting ourselves some slack also means being more content with our lot, as this brings freedom.

While imprisoned in Rome, St Paul wrote:

> I know what it is to be in need, and I know what it is to have plenty. I have learned the secret of being content in any and every situation, whether well fed or hungry, whether living in plenty or in want.

Contentment is not about denying our feelings, it is about accepting them for what they are, rather than a measure of ourselves and our value.

Discontentment drives us to want more stuff, exotic experiences, fancy food, none of which – as we know well – will bring us long-term satisfaction but disappointment, self-judgement, and even shame. We relate better to ourselves when we are content with what we have and our situation, and are compassionate with ourselves. In turn, we relate better to other people.

Self-contentment also means being easier on ourselves when things do not go as well as they might have; it also enables us to place more appropriate emphasis on spending time building our own resilience.

Be honest with yourself

The big question is to be asking whether we are doing our best given the whole situation, and being honest with ourselves. Self-discipline is about doing the things we need to do when we don't feel like it. Self-compassion is being realistic about how much of each we can actually do, and facing up to ourselves with honesty and humility.

Do you do your best? If you don't try as hard as you could, is that because of some mitigating factor rather than a real or imagined personality defect? Focusing on the level of effort invested in a task or activity releases us from results obsession, and therefore frees us up for greater self-compassion.

Building compassion for ourselves has a virtual cycle with our compassion for others. The Bible tells us in Galatians 5:22–23 that 'the fruit of the Spirit is love, joy, peace, long-suffering, kindness, goodness, faithfulness, gentleness and self-control'. Notice how the first four of these are inner 'fruits' which, when developed within us, lead to the growth and production of the other five. So, loving yourself like you do your pet or an elderly relative will build your resilience for the future, as well as that of other people; while providing a benchmark for those times when, despite everything we do, it all goes awry.

The well-known poem 'Desiderata' by Max Ehrmann says it all better than I could possibly hope to do. There's a link to the poem in the Reading list on page 186, so please take a moment to read what he says.

Next steps

1. Where are you being overly harsh or judgemental on yourself? Be careful that you are listening to a supportive and encouraging inner voice.
2. What do you have to do to give yourself permission for a time out to work all of this through?
3. Read the 'Desiderata' and reflect on the area(s) in life for which you need to practise creating contentment. What will that mean you accepting or giving up?

21. Recuperation, rest and sleep

> 'Our minds must have relaxation: rested, they will rise up better and keener. Just as we must not force fertile fields (for uninterrupted production will quickly exhaust them), so continual labor will break the power of our minds. They will recover their strength, however, after they have had a little freedom and relaxation.'
>
> Seneca

Recuperation

Discovering that creative practice aids recovery from traumatic events may go some way to explaining why Winston Churchill spent a lot of his spare time creating more than 500 paintings. You may not have developed such painting skills, but 'creative' does not have to mean fine art. It could be something as simple as letting your inner child out through using nature to create something in the style of artist Andy Goldsworthy, model-making, playing some music or writing poetry.

Taking creative time out can give you space to think and feel through past events, as can involvement in the arts in general. Interactions with animals and physical activity are now well known to be beneficial by providing a sense of purpose and meaning. Art therapy in particular has been found to be very beneficial in developing resilience for when adversity strikes. (Kelly, 2012 and Mudaly, et al., 2012)

One simple way of accessing these benefits can be to use the modern adult colouring books. Many people find these helpful in managing stress or anxiety because the precision of physical action required is completely absorbing – similar to the effect a run of more than 30 minutes or climbing, as described earlier. It seems that by focusing on physical activity, our mental activities are realised from prior constraints and able to run free. Taking this one step further, activities that align with our communication preference also may enable this 'switch'. If you would rather try creating images than colouring in, you could try something inspired by the Zentangle® method of pattern drawing. This art technique is easy to learn, very absorbing and satisfying. Here is one of mine (Figure 8).

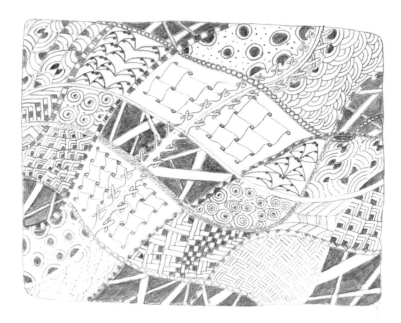

Figure 8: Zentangle drawing

'In drawing you delve deeply into a part of your mind too often obscured by endless details of daily life... Creative solutions to problems, whether personal of professional, will be accessible through new modes of thinking and new ways of using the power of your whole brain.'

(Edwards, 1992)

Learning to draw can help you to learn how to switch between logical thinking and creative thinking, which then becomes easier to achieve in other contexts.

Your recuperation may not be art-based, but this is another area where a little experimentation is necessary. One senior police officer I know spends some of their weekends as a volunteer on a steam railway, shovelling coal into the heat of the furnace. It is so completely different to their day job that it has recuperating effects.

While recuperation should be a part of our daily lives, it is even more important to include after a challenging event.

The Post-Incident Management (PIM) process used widely in UK police forces is designed to facilitate investigation into an incident and ensure the welfare of the staff and officers involved. As PIM requires those involved to provide a written record of events soon afterwards, it has the effect of causing them to reflect as well. The Trauma Risk Management (TRiM) process goes further, in that it aims to identify and manage the welfare needs of the individuals involved in a traumatic process – including signposting them to specialist medical care, and can include some kind of personal journalling. The psychologist James W. Pennebaker has shown that journalling our deepest thoughts and feelings about a situation can improve not only mental but physical health.

Returning to a purely physical situation, consider the marathon runner. It is not unusual to find going downstairs very difficult the day after a race. Therefore, trying to go out for a run is out of the question: this is obvious because of the physical pain. Shouldn't we be allowing for mental recovery from challenging times too?

Rest versus sleep

'Rest time is not waste time. It is economy to gather fresh strength... It is wisdom to take occasional furlough. In the long run, we shall do more by sometimes doing less.'

Charles Spurgeon

Rest is the one thing that the modern life of busyness has robbed us of, mostly without our noticing. 'Having a rest' is now almost a parallel to being lazy, a slacker or worse still, not committed. Yet we know intuitively when we should rest and, as Spurgeon says, it gives us 'fresh strength'.

There was a time when large corporates, universities and even churches allowed staff to take a sabbatical from their work. Some used the space to write books, visit and work in other parts of the world; in the case of missionaries, when it was referred to as furlough, return to their home countries to catch up with family and friends and recharge.

True rest is that which sees you lose track of time, and return to the human being that you really are. Outwardly it may look somewhat pointless, yet inwardly it is invaluable.

Canvas recharging

For several years when our children were much younger, we took our holidays camping. From wind-swept sites on clifftops in West Wales to tranquil lakeside pine groves on small Canadian islands, life adopted a slower more relaxed and natural pace. The children from across the site seemed to congregate under our canvas during the days, all contentedly playing or chatting together. There was little purpose other than to just be. Eating when hungry, sleeping when it was too dark to read.

Watching the sun go down, the clouds in the sky, hearing the breeze through the trees are all inherently restful and recharge our depleted souls. We all know how beneficial this is for us, yet the only time we allow for it is on holiday while, actually, we would benefit from building an element of it into everyday life.

If we know the benefits, why are we not making more room for it? My hunch is not just that it is seen as 'weak' or even childish, but that we have allowed technology to rob us of the space. It isn't just the TV – it is our 'always-on' attitude and – more importantly – the ease with which we can entertain ourselves in that downtime: whether that is Instagram, YouTube, TED, Pinterest or any of the social media platforms. There is undoubtedly a close connection between the paucity of our rest and our lack of margin allowance and lack of boundaries. It is time to just stand there, instead of doing something. Rest and mindfulness are closely connected, as long as we are not trying so hard.

If there were one thing worth exploring, it would be restoring a day of rest for ourselves. Free of digital devices, maybe TV and definitely shopping. It may cost you a little to get your food shop delivered, but the rest you could get instead would have a value far in excess. Rest allows for recovery as much as rebuilding for the next event that life will serve up. As Ovid, the Roman poet (43 BC to AD 17), said: 'Take rest: a field that has rested gives a beautiful crop.'

Sleep

> 'Sleep is the single most effective thing we can do to reset our brain and body health each day.'
>
> (Walker, 2018)

In the last three years there has been an explosion in the number of books about sleep. This section will not repeat them, simply highlight some of the key points.

What is interesting is not that this is suddenly an area of interest; but more that we need any books at all. We inherently know that we need to sleep, and that we suffer when we don't. What we did not know until now is why. Previously, sleep – or more accurately, not sleeping – had become a macho, tough thing: something we should need less of. What we have learned now is that reducing our sleep, whether purposefully or otherwise, has seriously negative impacts on our immune system and physical and mental health.

Sleep is tied to our overall health to such a great extent that, if it were possible to create any other mechanisms to achieve the same result, we would all be willing to pay for it. The irony is, of course, that this magical health promoting process is actually free (unless you want to put a cost on the things that you might have to give up in order to achieve it).

Four things seem key in this regard – think CATS: caffeine, alcohol, technology and sunset.

Caffeine

> **Nick was right!**
>
> I went through a long patch of poor sleep, and my friend Nicholas regularly asked me about my coffee-drinking habits. I consistently denied that the two were in any way related – mainly because I was not drinking a vast quantity, and my problem was not going to sleep; it was waking up during the night and lying awake for hours.

It turns out that this uncontrolled, addictive substance has far more impact on us than I had imagined before researching this book. The most telling example was an experiment done in 1948 by a Swiss pharmacologist named Peter N. Witt who studied the effects of caffeine and psychotic drugs on the ability of spiders to create a web.

While cannabis resulted in a more accurate spider's web, others had a more negative effect – and caffeine was the worst of all. The webs were random and basically useless. While we should take care in extrapolating from arachnid to human; it seems most unlikely that there would be no parallels.

According to Walker, Caffeine operates by blocking the receptors in our brain for the hormone adenosine, which makes us feel tired. Tiredness continues to build, and caffeine just stops it being effective until it wears off anything between 5 and 7 hours later. This is what gives us that crashing tiredness late in the day – which we often overcome with another double-shot espresso. That may keep you awake long into the night, resulting in groggy tiredness the next day – which, of course, we self-medicate with even more coffee, and so on.

Decaffeinated coffee is slightly better, but still contains around one-quarter of the normal amount of caffeine. Since reading about this negative cycle I have avoided the dreaded stuff after 12 pm each day, and now sleep noticeably better. Nicholas turned out to be right after all!

Alcohol

Many of us have experienced the impact that alcohol has on us. While everyone is affected differently and to greater or lesser extent, alcohol acts to remove certain inhibitions and appears to help us sleep well. However, that is not true, as alcohol is a *sedative*. The sedative effect removes our inhibitions and knocks us out, but that is also why, after one too many drinks, we fall asleep quickly and wake almost as quickly a few hours later. We feel bad and have been 'asleep' – yet it is not sleep, it is sedation.

The tiredness remains, so when we finally wake up after a disturbed night, we feel bad. Yes, the hangover may be due to dehydration, but it is perfectly possible to wake up in precisely the same state without any alcohol at all (as many who have been through the toddler years of constantly interrupted sleep can confirm). Impaired ability after a night out and too many glasses of wine is probably as much to do with tiredness as the inhibitory function of the alcohol. Indeed, it seems that going without sleep for more than 19 hours can have the same effect without any alcohol at all.

It is also important to consider that because alcohol impacts the early hours of sleep, our ability to solidify new learning is reduced. Students and those trying to learn new skills and facts, take note!

Technology

It is now well understood that the plethora of LED illumination around us and the blue light that it creates have a negative impact on our sleep. The problem is, these things are now everywhere: TVs, light bulbs, tablets, smartphones, ebook readers, even bathroom cabinet lighting. Exposing ourselves to this wavelength of blue light blocks the natural increase in melatonin in our bloodstream, which in turn delays feelings of tiredness, and makes it harder to fall asleep. It also reduces the type of sleep that we need to integrate learning and control our emotions. (Of course, we can use this to our advantage by getting plenty of blue-light early in the day to wake ourselves up! – I routinely turn the bathroom cabinet lights on first thing now.)

Newer smartphones and tablets now have features built-in to shift the colour temperature to 'warmer' – less blue, and more yellow at either set times or at dusk and sunrise. (It is possible that, while manufacturers want us to see them as having a social conscience, this was actually done so that we would continue using these attention-trapping beasts longer into the night.) Beware that older tablets and mobile phones may not have this feature.

Apart from the light effects of our PDAs, there is also the impact of the actual content that we are consuming. Endless social media and email threads read late at night often end up circulating around in our minds as we are trying to get to sleep, keeping us awake unnecessarily. So move the TV out of the bedroom, leave the laptop, tablet and phone outside, and get a proper old-fashioned alarm clock instead!

Sunset

Given all these factors, it would be worth experimenting with developing a sunset routine – a window of time before we retire to bed during which we dim the lights (or turn a lot of them off), avoid our electronics and perhaps have a warm bath or shower and read a real book in bed with a cup of herbal tea, having made the bedroom cool and dark.

What if you still can't go to sleep, even after all this? Try getting up and writing a stream-of-consciousness to get your thoughts down on paper, with a pen. Bed should be reserved for sleeping and sex, rather than TVs and tablets.

The same goes for the middle of the night, when it is very likely your animal brain and its inner voice are worrying and muttering in your ear. Don't ruminate, just write it down. Lying in bed awake for more than 15 minutes only extends the wakefulness – so go to the bathroom, write down the murmurations in your head, then return to bed, turn over and let yourself fall asleep.

No amount of trying will help you with a sleep problem, but these things just might. If they don't, go and see a doctor – they will not just give you pills! It does seem that one of the problems with knowing how important sleep is to us can result in anxiety about sleeping. (Think back to the night before having to get up early to travel, or an interview.)

Don't just lie there, do something!

Next steps

1. If you have a sleeping difficulty, please consider getting some medical advice
2. Build times of rest into every day, especially after significant events. If relevant, find out who runs the PIM, TRiM, or similar process in your organisation.
3. Choose an activity that you can use as recuperation, and plan time in your day and/or week to do it.
4. Decide on a sunset routine, put it into practice for 28 days and journal what happens.

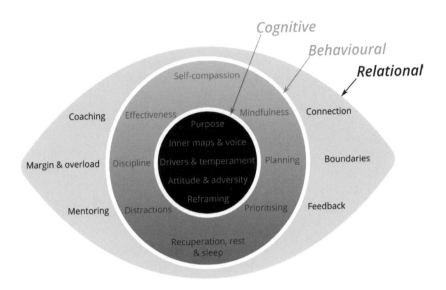

Part 4: Relational factors

> 'Overload is not having time to finish the book you're reading...
> Margin is having time to read it twice. Margin is the space that once
> existed between ourselves and our limits.'
>
> (Swenson, 2004)

Margin is that space around the edge of the page that we leave. When we were at school, it was to give the teacher space to add comments and marks. On a book such as this, it enables you to hold it without covering up the text, or even annotate it with your own thoughts.

Whatever business sector you consider, whether private or public, it seems that we are experiencing an overload epidemic: whether it be volume of work, choice, change, fatigue or expectation, overload is everywhere we turn.

In the early days of industrialisation, predictions were that by the 20th and 21st century people would have an abundance of free time due to the efficiencies provided by automation and labour-saving equipment – but we seem to have gone in the opposite direction. What we have gained instead of free time is overload.

Margin is the gap between the resources we have available (including energy, skills, finances, etc.) and consumption (e.g. work volume and expectations; problems; personal expectations; deadlines etc.). More succinctly, $M = R - C$.

How lack of margin affects us

A lack of margin in our lives causes us to suffer in a variety of ways: it steals the rest that we so badly need. We attempt to address our suffering through medication and/or wellbeing programmes, whereas a more useful solution might be to create more margin instead – more time to breathe, think and recuperate.

The big problem with overload caused by lack of margin is that we cannot see it coming, and it can be upon us before we are aware of what is really happening. Sometimes we are lucky enough to have a partner, family or friends who can spot it earlier than we do, but in my experience, we often deny being stressed instead of taking action.

Margin gives us greater capacity in all areas of our lives: relational, spiritual, emotional and physical. Time margin, or the lack thereof, is widely prevalent in our language today. We talk of having 'no time', 'not enough time', 'lack of time', 'time being of the essence', and even 'managing time' – what a misnomer that is! We need to shift this language towards *growing* our time margin, perhaps by talking instead of 'time together', 'family time', 'quiet time', 'prayer time', or 'thinking time'.

Without margin, these are the kind of activities we drop to the bottom of our priority list because we think of them as discretionary and 'nice to have'. They are clearly no such thing – they are essential to a fulfilling life. We should be actively creating more time margin by allowing for and expecting interruptions or disruptions, growing the strength of our 'no', and pruning our diaries.

Margin leading to customer delight

It is likely that at some point, you will have travelled on a budget airline. One in particular, EasyJet, seems to manage better than the others, to be on time. Amazingly, even though a recent flight I took to Belfast departed late, it still landed on time. Nothing to do with a tailwind, as the journey is too short for that to have a significant positive impact.

This is all down to leaving a bit of margin. After all, when you fly half a million sectors a year from 132 airports, you tend to learn where delays are most likely to happen, so you can make adjustments and build in margin. The load may change unexpectedly, but over the course of time, EasyJet has got better at predicting what is going to go wrong, and expanded the 'power' in the system to provide more margin – which in turn delights customers like me!

Open an emotional bank account

Diary pruning will release time that we then can use to create further margin in the areas of our physical and emotional life, so that instead of being overwhelmed and under-rested we are able to keep in better health, as well as enjoying another significant benefit.

The principle of the 'emotional bank account' (EBA – as introduced in Chapter 17) is one I learned over than 20 years ago on a leadership course in my early days at Hewlett-Packard. The idea is that by meeting our commitments to others and going the extra mile, we make a 'deposit' into an imaginary account of emotional commitment to us by the other person. The result of building up this kind of 'credit' is that when we do not meet our commitments or we forget meetings, then our relationship can survive – at least for a time.

It never occurs to any of us to ask about our own EBA. While the things we personally value are different, some of us live with our EBA in the black, while others hover perilously close to the red line – and when we cross it, we are the ones who suffer, along with those closest to us.

Fortunately there are several ways to make a deposit into our personal EBA through rest and recuperation, as well as the obvious ones of socialising, laughter, grace, gratitude and paying it forward. Even getting clear on our purpose can improve our emotional margin by increasing our EBA.

More room to breathe

Mark is a senior police officer who kept finding himself trapped without time to get lunch, or being late for meetings. When we explored the true situation by looking at his calendar, the thing that jumped out was that most of his meetings were back-to-back. Even those requiring travel sometimes did not allow any time for transition, let alone something realistic. There was no margin in his diary. So, if one meeting overran, then the whole day was late.

Mark decided on a slightly unusual course of action: he shortened all the meetings he leads to 45 minutes, while continuing to start them on the hour or half-hour. He also asked his personal assistant to allow a 10 per cent margin on all his travel time between meetings, if necessary. The upside? He now has room to breathe. Room to be mindful. Room to stop and reflect how events are unfolding, and thus have a greater sense of control. He even has room for a sociable lunch occasionally!

Creating margin in our lives emotionally, physically, spiritually and in how we spend our time is surely better than 'just hanging in there for the next 3 years until I retire', as someone said to me recently.

Next steps

1. Check your calendar for margin. Do you have back-to-back meetings? How can you increase your margin each day?

2. Start planning time in for margin allowance in the same way as a project manager allows for delays in their project.

3. Who do you need to bring on-side to create margin for both of you?

23. Boundaries

Identifying boundaries

By identifying boundaries we create limits between the different areas of our life to stop the world invading it uninvited. This is as much about self-care as anything else: other people will violate your boundaries if you allow them to do so. Once is probably enough to get you taking up the slack and turning their emergency into yours again and again. Why do we do this? You will have your own reasons – often it is about wanting to be helpful or seen as reliable, dependable and a safe pair of hands.

Apparently, when asked if he would take something on, Nobel-prize winning physicist Richard Feynman would say he was irresponsible: 'If anybody asks me to be on a committee to take care of admissions, "No, I'm irresponsible. I don't give a damn about the students." Of course I give a damn about the students, but I know that somebody else'll do it.' Isn't it time that you stopped taking on others' tasks by setting clearer boundaries for yourself?

This is not about becoming unhelpful and refusing to go the extra mile or more; rather, making a conscious decision about when to say 'no' and when to say 'yes' – and once you have decided, you must *own* it.

If it is true that we spend only 2 per cent of our time thinking about other people, then it is very unlikely that they will hold it against us for long – if at all. Practising setting better boundaries gives you the best opportunities to do those things that build resilience for the future. This does require us to know what is and is not part of our job, as when we routinely take on tasks that are not really ours, eventually we will pay the price with exhaustion and burnout.

There are four key types of boundaries to consider:

- Physical

- Emotional
- Mental
- Spiritual

We need to know what our responsibilities are in each of these areas.

We all understand the principles of boundaries. We all face different challenges, of course, but when we fail to set clear boundaries with other people, or our families, we all suffer.

Spotify got them into trouble

Imagine a teenager with poor boundary management in terms of money. When you bail them out for the nth time, you effectively tell them that you will take on the negative outcome rather than let them take on their suffering.

When we first moved our teenagers on to phone contracts, within the space of a month they both racked up large data bills. Looking in detail, we found Spotify to be the cause and told them what to do about it and that they now would be responsible for the bill if they exceeded their data allowance.

It has not happened again – yet! Crossing that particular boundary again will give them a problem, not me.

Clarity on what is and is not ours sets us free, rather than straitjacketing us. Within our boundaries, we are free to do as we wish. However, this goes beyond our mental boundaries to our physical situation and words.

The importance of setting boundaries

There are times when physically avoiding a place – or extricating ourselves from one – sets a boundary and allows us either to avoid a situation, or create one that is more calming. This may be challenging for you: for example, a job in a caring profession can seem to be at odds with setting boundaries.

Perhaps it is more helpful to think about the consequences of boundary violation as if it were trespassing. Fences are there to stop people (and animals) from entering a space uninvited. Work-life boundaries have a similar purpose. The consequences to us of work-life trespassing are that we make commitments under pressure and/or give in to the demands placed on us by other people, when deep down in our heart of hearts we know we should not. Maybe we need to worry less about people not loving our 'no' as much as our 'yes'?

All behaviours have consequences – for those behaving as much as those on the receiving end. We all need to take more responsibility for our choices, especially in high-volume, high-pressure jobs. When we say 'yes' too many times, we often end up regretting it eventually.

In the same way that we cannot change others, only ourselves, we cannot impose boundaries on them. It is not just about the difficulty in saying 'no' though. Sometimes learning that it is bad to say 'no' can result in allowing others to treat us as they wish. This becomes more significant when we encounter someone who is manipulative or controlling.

If you are finding it hard to say 'no', is it because you fear a negative outcome, e.g. punishment, career limitations, perception, anger? If so, consider the evidence of the likelihood of that, as well as the potential cost. It could be that creating a boundary by clearly saying 'no' will be more positive than negative – especially if you take a long-term view.

Realisation from proper recuperation

Luke is pretty fit and active, but got the flu last winter, and it took weeks to recover. Eventually he was signed off sick from work and had to rest completely. Nothing unusual in that story – we all know folk who have had a similar experience.

What makes it interesting is that he says he now realises how unimportant some of the things were that he was worrying about trying to do, instead of recuperating. He has decided to share his view, do the best he can and create clearer boundaries in his life, between work and family, and times of play and rest.

Your boundaries define what you have decided to exert power over – namely, what falls inside. Everything else falls outside, by definition. This in turn helps us to keep short accounts with ourselves, instead of blaming ourselves when things don't go as well as they could have.

The key is to remember that *in any relationship, the only thing we can change is how we perceive and respond to the other person.* So when someone else's actions are destructive to us, we need to change how we deal with them, so that they are no longer destructive. This calls for wisdom: that of knowing what is and isn't ours. What's inside and outside our boundaries.

If you are worried that setting boundaries will make you seem selfish or disobedient, consider that a lack of boundaries is more likely to *lead to* selfish or disobedient behaviour, because inwardly we feel resentful, and that inward 'no' cannot be made up for by yet another external 'yes'. Our thoughts, beliefs and values are inextricably linked to our actions and results, as we have seen already. So when we mean 'no' but say 'yes', the internal 'no' will only create a poorer end result. It also may create a resentment that builds over time only to explode later, creating a much worse net result.

Taking on too much work is a very similar problem, and needs to be addressed in a similar manner. Don't let someone with poor boundaries force you to do the same, or to violate yours. This is just taking the monkey off their back and putting it onto your own. Let them keep the monkey. No doubt you have quite enough monkeys of your own.

Whether it is about your diary or something else, some advice I was given early in my consulting career might be useful:

> People will ask you for a discount and say things about their budget, or that they can buy your service cheaper elsewhere. First, that's a lie – only you can sell your service, by definition. Second, if they want to pay less, you simply ask which part of the service they don't want! *Decide your boundaries, practise the words if necessary, and stick to them.*

A lot of bosses do not realise how lucky they are: their staff take the responsibility for their lack of planning and never impose any limits back, violating their own boundaries and leading to burnout. The net result is that the boss loses a key staff member, probably much to their surprise. But not to yours now, I hope.

So, we need to set clearer boundaries on things like:

- what is and isn't our work
- how much (and how often) we will do overtime
- our personal lives

– all of which we will maintain fiercely and graciously. This requires us to know our physical, mental, spiritual and emotional limits, and to prioritise their maintenance.

Going outside the boundaries of your work can only mean breaking the boundaries of your non-work life. So when you feel that your work-related stress is impacting your non-working life, evaluate which boundaries are being violated and take steps, with help if necessary, to reinforce them – just as you would fix a fence to keep the fox from your chickens, the deer off your roses, and so on.

Boundaries and margin are closely coupled, in that margin is the space that falls just inside the boundary. Practically, this means that you need clarity on your boundaries just as much as you need to allow margin. Together, this pair form an essential part of creating a resilient life and working environment.

Next steps
1. How clearly have you defined the boundaries between what is and isn't work for you? What could they be, and which are most important to you?
2. Think about situations when you might need to cross them, and how you can limit the frequency of such 'trespassing'.

24. Physical environment

'Our environment is a non-stop triggering mechanism while impact on our behaviour is too significant to be ignored.'

(Goldsmith, 2016)

Clear your space

The outer environment within which we live and move has a greater impact on our inner life than we might think. Imagine a room – maybe your garage or a shed – that is filled with stuff that needs sorting out. Every time you enter it, part of you is embarrassed or even ashamed that you cannot sort it out. This is referred to as an 'open loop' – an unresolved situation or question.

Open loops can suck the energy from us, cause us to worry, ruminate and even lose sleep. Just think about how it feels while you wait to hear about some test results. A good GP surgery will phone to let you know, even if the results are clear – such is the burden of the open loop. So you shut the door of the shed to put it out of your mind, in an attempt to close the loop.

A pile of boxes

I attended a webinar recently where an audience member described how she had a pile of unopened moving boxes in her lounge, despite having moved in more than a year earlier. Rather than unpack or move them, she covered them with a cloth and put screens around them when people came to visit. She added that whenever she looked at the cloth or the screens, something 'kind of dies inside me'.

It is not just a whole room, sometimes it is just the space in which we work. As the old saying goes, 'A tidy desk shows a tidy mind' (to which I used to flippantly respond 'or someone who is not really working at all').

Our response to what happens to us are impacted as much by the environment in which they happen as how we think about them. It can be far easier to change the environment than our thinking – especially if speed is of the essence.

Deliberately anchor yourself

Another key thing about environment is that we tend to psychologically associate specific places with specific activities. Think about a meeting that you attend regularly, and notice that for the most part, you – and everyone else – always take the same seat. We are all creatures of habit, after all. If you have ever had a visitor who sits in 'someone else's' usual seat, you will have noticed that there is a subtle shift in the dynamic in the room. Sometimes I will deliberately sit where someone else normally does, in order to trigger such changes. With this in mind, it might be worth getting people to regularly move around, especially if discussions are becoming static.

From a resilience perspective, we can use this 'anchoring' behaviour to our advantage: for example, by choosing a particular place to go to relax (maybe the floor of the gym), a particular chair or coffee shop, if that is possible. If you repeatedly carry out the daily reflection that we covered in Part 3 in the same place, it will become increasingly easier to do.

Other things that are part of the environment include the lighting, colours, background noise and music. If you have ever been on a long train journey and lucky enough to have a table to sit at, you might have noticed that you think more creatively and (other passengers permitting) are able to concentrate and get a lot more done than you usually would. While that may be partly to do with a lack of other distractions and interruptions, apparently the colours of the world outside also help. It is not referred to as blue-sky thinking by accident!

All of these things are triggers, stimulants almost, in our environment that we can use to positively influence our state, our ability to concentrate, and so on.

There are also triggers that come from our environment which negatively impact our resilient state and willpower. Environment can be part of the reason why we do not make the changes we seek, and so it is one of the first places to start when we want a change that really sticks – even just a simple one.

Reducing the cognitive load

Writing this at my desk today, there is a pile of pens and pencils to my right, the draft copies of the text to my left, a couple of books I have referred to for quotes, my phone and an almost empty cup of stone cold tea. Charging cables, headphones and notebooks are spread around me.

> While the software I am using fills the screen, a calendar reminder has just popped up. Every single piece of this is crowding into my brain for attention. All trying to get on the stage of my mind, while I battle to keep it off.
>
> Let's clear it for a moment… and breathe.
>
> Now that the things on the desk are only those that I need, I am typing noticeably faster. I have reduced the cognitive load, so it feels easier too.

Consider your online environment – whether that is via a browser or an app such as Instagram (which is actually just a fancy kind of browser) – especially apps such as these, which have design features to keep your interest in the same way that a supermarket or casino is designed to prise money from you.

How do we avoid them? If it is the casino, that is easy – just don't go through the doors. The supermarket? By not walking up and down every aisle that you know you have no need of – which will require a shopping list, and sticking to it! All of these are about having a deliberate outcome.

Design your environment

What outcome have you designed your environment to produce? You may not have done it deliberately, but you have done it all the same. This is a type of feedback too: the environment triggers your behaviour, and thus your results. If the results are not what you want, then it is worth going back to the beginning and working out what they are, then deciding how to change the environment to achieve them. Create multiple different ones, if you wish. With a bit of thought and regular use, you can create a virtuous loop where just entering the environment triggers the behaviour you want.

> ### Use music to trigger a state
>
> For the last six months I have been applying the discipline of weekly planning as the first thing I do on Monday mornings.
>
> The first step is to clear the desk, get the planner out, and listen to Beethoven's *Pastoral Symphony*. The first couple of bars alone are now enough to shift my thinking into planning mode, and I have usually finished by the time the symphony reaches its finale.

Taking the time to build an environment which triggers the behaviours you want when you are not in a crisis, will help to build your resilience for when you need do it later. While you cannot always control the environment around you, especially in challenging situations, awareness of how it is influencing you, and making small changes, can help you to be more resilient.

Next steps

1. What do you think your environment is triggering in your behaviour today? What could be better than that? How can you change it to achieve the results you really want?
2. Which environments in your life sap your energy? Are they open loops such as those described? What could you change to close them?
3. Consider creating an environment (physical and/or virtual) that will quickly enable you to return to a resilient and resourceful state. What would that be like? (For example, think about a rich sensory experience.)

25. Connection

'*Abihaze ham ntakibanariva* – Nothing can defeat combined hands.'

Rwandan

Our culture seems to place too high a value on our work and careers, often at the expense of our relationships. Yet we were made for connection, for relationships, for one another.

Just think of the things that have brought you deepest joy. Most likely they involve other people. A shared, challenging experience is one that often creates bonds of friendship that survive for decades. Where times of separation simply melt away when we meet again – that is why we have reunions. Well, that is the hope behind them; sadly, often they can descend into subtle (or not-so-subtle) one-upmanship.

When we spend time together and have the right attitude (or mindset), we can increase our resilience. I have been running workshops covering a variety of topics with UK police forces for the last seven years, and one of the most common reflections on feedback forms is: 'I now realise that I am not alone.' We think that we are the only ones who find our email overwhelming, or the challenges of balancing family life with work, or just simply getting out of bed to face yet another day on the front line. If only we were to build and maintain stronger, more open connections with one another, we would realise that everyone else is struggling with something of which we are utterly unaware.

Isn't this what makes little children so charming – as well as simultaneously embarrassing – at times? They say what they see, and what they think. But as we grow up, we learn the cultural norms as to what is and is not appropriate to say. However, many of today's issues come from some people feeling that it is fine to remove their 'inappropriateness' filters online: maybe we are finding out what we are really like, and finally seeing the depth of our depravity?

The real downside of all this filtering is that we are trying to protect ourselves, to make ourselves appear OK. We don't ask people to help us 'because they already have a lot on', or 'I don't want to be a bother'. We should ask more often, rather than less – and at the same time, give one another permission to decline. We need to grow our 'no'.

I've got too much else on

My son is a keen hockey player, so I spend a lot of time watching matches. After one game, a club committee member approached me and asked if I would be able to help organise the team for the season:

'Nothing much, just getting the names of who's available and letting people know when and where matches are, that kind of thing.'

Now, I could have done it – I am not bad at organising people, and I was pleased to be asked. But I challenged my inner dialogue that, if I am honest, said: 'Ooo, he's asking *me* to help! I can do that. That would be helpful.' (I sometimes think I was brought up believing helpfulness is close to godliness.)

But I said: 'No, sorry. I've got too much else on.'
'Oh, OK, no problem – just thought I'd ask.'
We are still friends, and I don't think he thinks ill of me.

The problem is that as our connectedness has weakened, we have stopped treating one another as adults, and now we make decisions for one another without actually asking. All coming from a place of kindness – but actually disempowering one another.

How to connect well

What do we need to have better connections? Openness about how our lives really are. About what we observe going on in one another's lives. In fact, to be even more *involved* in each other's lives. By this, I do not mean just having friends round to dinner every so often, or going on an annual weekend trip. I mean the down-to-earth, daily stuff.

Maybe you are a member of a sports club, arts club or drama group, so you know something of this. These are places where a plumber may participate alongside a police officer, an administrator alongside an actuary, a graphic designer alongside a gardener. You share a common interest in the activity, and as you do that, you share your lives with one another. But sadly, this is so often just at arm's length.

Getting to know one another better and sharing our lives means that when life does get difficult, we have people whom we can trust and share our challenges with, knowing that they will not judge us but will help us as they feel able, even if it is just to listen. The real tragedy of the mental health crisis in our society seems to be best summed up by: 'If only they had talked to someone.'

We all realise now that social media such as Facebook, Instagram or Twitter are broadcast media. They may have started out as a way to share our lives, but as the number of adverts continues to rise, they are less inherently social. It is like going to the annual school reunion where no one is real about their lives, just constantly elevating themselves or diminishing someone else. Worse still, these applications are designed to suck our attention and retain it: there are no obvious signposts to stop, so we spend our 'relational time' there instead of actually talking to people. What a waste of time.

'Where there is no sharing, there can be no friendship. Wise men say... that heaven and earth, gods and men, are held together by the principles of sharing, by friendship and order, by self-control and justice.'

Socrates

Next steps

1. How much time are you spending on an electronic device instead of building true relationships? What can you do to change that, either by revitalising old friendships or building new ones around a shared interest?

2. Who do you need to give permission to be completely open and honest with you, and yourself with them?

26. Feedback

> 'You only live one life, and you make all your mistakes, and learn what not to do, and that's the end of you.'
>
> Richard Feynman

The word 'feedback', more than almost any other, can push even the most fearless and confident person into a tailspin. The problem is that giving feedback is routinely done extremely badly. However, when done well, it can help us all to become more aware of where we can increase our performance and resilience, and where it is already strong.

Recent research shows that regular feedback is one of the best ways to retain, develop and improve the engagement of staff. Over the last few years, several large multinational corporations have introduced formal feedback and coaching programmes in lieu of annual performance reviews (which one found to have contributed precisely $0 to their bottom-line results). (Kaye and Jordan-Evans, 2005)

The 'feedback sandwich'

The most common method of giving feedback has been to use the 'feedback sandwich' – where you mention the thing that someone does badly between two positive comments. But it is loathsome, and it does not work. It should have been consigned to the Room 101 of management tools aeons ago. Why? Consider these two examples:

- Someone who has been in a tailspin all day, waiting for their feedback, does not even hear the first bit (that is, if they don't just ignore it as being patronising), and may focus so much on the 'filling' that they never hear the final positive either. So they walk away feeling flattened.
- Some people only recall the final thing they heard, and walk out of your carefully planned session having completely missed the 'filling', believing things are perfectly OK as they are – no changes required.

I used to teach another feedback model as part of an Institute of Leadership (ILM) coaching and mentoring course. I could never remember it, even after several deliveries. So I looked for a better one.

From listening to hundreds of workshop participants, I have found that the problems with most feedback include:

- It is overly personal.
- It is vague – lacking concrete information.
- The person delivering it has an agenda.
- There is no room for discussion – often because there are no facts.
- It lacks direction – what could be changed or repeated.
- It is third-hand.
- It is too long after the event.
- There is no follow-up.

A NICER way to feed back

So I came up with another, which addresses all the above concerns: The NICER feedback model:

N – I Noticed

I – the Impact was

C – Check (did you notice too?), and then Change (if there is something to be changed) and/or Continue (if there is something that would be good to do again next time)

E – Effect (the future effect will be)

R – Review

If you are a trained coach, then you could replace the 'C' step with the word 'Coaching'.

A simple example would be:

'I noticed that you were very quiet in the team meeting today, which meant that we didn't hear your great ideas on [X]. Can I just check, is there anything wrong that I can help with…?

What would be good next time is to speak up – you have some great ideas which we need…

The effect of doing that will be to accelerate our progress…

Are you OK if we check in again after next week's meeting?'

The beauty of this model, participants say, is that it:

- is fast – you can deliver something meaningful and useful in just a few sentences, if you do not have much time
- is easy to remember

- covers the key areas
- can be used to give as well as get.

So the next time you are tempted to send an email saying something like 'Nice job over the weekend', you can pause and do a NICER job. You will find that you get an even better result next time. If you get such an email, then it is easy to respond with:

> 'Many thanks for your feedback. Can you just tell me what you noticed I did, and the effect that this had?
> Is there anything that I should avoid doing, as well as make sure I do again next time? What effect do you think and hope it will have in the future?'

Overall, this has to be nicer than a feedback sandwich.

With our focus here being more on building resilience than leadership development, the real value of feedback is getting an external view on how we are doing. So it is closely linked with the previous ingredient of reflection. If we are to be balanced in our self-awareness, we need both.

Without repercussions

Can you get fired for asking why?

After publishing an article on growth mindset in a UK policing magazine, I received a long email addressing what I had written about. Included in the message was this key point: 'Feedback needs to be taken both ways without repercussions.'

It reminded me of a workshop where I said: 'No one ever got fired for asking "why?", did they?' – and got the immediate response:

'They might not fire you, but they'll make sure you never get promoted.'

In old-style command-and-control organisations, the more senior you became, the less acceptable it was to be given feedback from those below you in the hierarchy. There is no place for this any more. As Commander L. David Marquet remarks in his excellent book, *Turn the Ship Around* (2012) (a great read as well as being one of the very best, if not *the* best, leadership book you will find), 'you have to push the responsibility down to where the information lies'.

By that, Marquet means that the people in your organisation who are at the coalface every day: whether that is dealing with members of the public or customers on the phone, *they* are the ones who really know what is going on. You may have done the exact same job, but unless you have walked alongside them for a few days in the last month (or even week, given the rate of change at present), then you cannot honestly say that you know what they are dealing with.

This is what makes coppers on the streets so frustrated when politicians make decisions that affect their day-to-day activities or terms of service. They are too remote and have no idea about the problem they are really solving, or the unforeseen consequences of the solution that they are pushing.

Instead, however senior you are within your force or organisation, can I encourage you to actively seek out feedback? I am sure there were times, when you were trying to get promoted, when you asked for candid feedback because you wanted to improve what you did, how you did it and your prospects too. Just because you do not want to climb further does not mean that you do not want to improve. So, give them permission to give you the feedback. Just have them do it in a NICER way!

Wherever we sit on an organisational chart, there is always room for us to do better.

Next steps
1. Practise the NICER feedback model, both in receiving as well as in giving.
2. Get some real feedback from your nearest and dearest about your resilience and what you might do to increase it, and in which areas.

27. Coaching and mentoring

'When given the opportunity to learn and grow, people thrive. By adopting a coaching mentality and approach, you can help members of your team realize their potential. An investment in employees will help retain top talent and foster a culture of growth and opportunity, which is a win for people and profit.'

Harvard

The review of resilience training programmes mentioned in Chapter 1 identified that there was wisdom, including some element of one-to-one and individual support in any programme, and hence its inclusion here.

It is clear that we cannot be resilient in all areas of our lives, just as much as we cannot always be resilient in the same areas all the time. Physical illness, for example, can reduce a previously highly physical resilient person for a while, but at the same time increase their capacity for learning – although we could argue that this in part is also a reflection of their mindset. Coaching can provide the support, challenge and accountability to get through a challenging situation and regain a sense of wellbeing.

Is it coaching or mentoring?

The terms *coaching* and *mentoring* seem to be used interchangeably, so for the avoidance of doubt, the definitions I use are as follows:

- A coach facilitates the coachee to explore their challenge, holding the belief that it is the coachee who has the best answers to their question. Consequently, the coach may better serve the relationship by having only an awareness of the context or challenge being explored. It can be more of a facilitation activity than a training one. The core ability that a coach must have is to be able to ask great questions.
- A mentor has deep experience in the context and/or challenge and provides guidance, solutions and answers to the challenges that the mentee faces. Having context-knowledge is an essential requirement of the mentor. A good mentor might employ coaching skills, while a coach might offer suggestions which the coachee can choose to hear and explore, or not.

Knowing when to occupy each role is crucial.

This is not a coaching opportunity

The first formal coaching training I attended was with David Hemery (400 m hurdles gold medallist in the 1968 Olympics). As a gifted athlete and coach, he gave me that initial spark to train as one myself.

To illustrate what coaching is and is not, he told us about when his son turned 18 and they went for their first driving lesson together. Sitting behind the wheel of the car for the first time, his son turned to him and said 'Dad. This is not a coaching opportunity.'

Coaching and mentoring have their place in building resilience. Indeed, those who both coach and mentor need a particular kind of resilience too: some coaches may see more than five clients a day, and need to have the resilience to keep their concentration up for the whole day.

Coaching can support building resilience in advance of an event, during one and (where appropriate) afterwards. It can provide a safe space to explore openly the facets of a situation which may have not been previously noticed, as well as opportunities not yet examined.

Depending on the coach's skill, they may be able to assist with reframing and other techniques already described. The key benefit that a coach can bring is being non-directive and having the ability to ask the obvious questions that someone with deep domain knowledge would not ask because of shared understanding. Not being 'in the know' turns out to be really helpful.

Not-knowing can be quicker

In my work with many police forces in the UK and Ireland, I have suggested frequently that I shadow someone in order to have a more in-depth understanding of the challenges they face. In one case, the response I got (even when I offered to do so without charge) was:

> That wouldn't be helpful. You *not* having understanding of the situation and *not* being security vetted means that the person

---

> talking to you is unable to give you the narrative, and thus you will get to the real heart of the issue faster.
>
> This has turned out to be true for more than one such engagement.

Coaching and mentoring can reinforce what has been learned in the training room – although again, with a slightly different approach. Coaching might start from exploring what has happened since the training, what worked and what has not, and so on; while mentoring might require something such as a written report as a starting point.

The main benefit of either approach is the one-to-one nature, as this provides the safety often required for people to really explore the boundaries of their approach and performance – and by doing so, provide a platform for real growth. Creating a coaching culture is another factor in making our organisations more resilient, even if it is only because people become more accustomed to talking about what is really happening for them.

The FLAME model

I have developed and used this model when working with middle and senior managers:

Feedback
Learning
Accountability
Mentoring
Encouragement

The point of the model is to provide a clear structure to coaching engagements.

Feedback

When we explore feedback together, the focus is on all of its types – as there is no situation in life when we are not receiving feedback. Sometimes there is external feedback, either written or spoken; while other times the most useful feedback is that gained from considering what keeps happening, or noticing that something has changed (either for the better or otherwise). Or it may be a repeating piece of dialogue from your inner voice.

Learning

As all feedback provides opportunities to learn (to believe so makes it so, of course!) we can then move to the 'Learning' phase. This could be from an external source (e.g. a training course, TED talk or book), or more internally as a result of reflection from feedback.

Accountability

Many of us need someone to be accountable to, but the higher we rise in our organisations, the less obvious it seems to be – and the more resistant we are to it, perhaps because we feel the need to appear to be 'on our A-game', or 'just cracking on with it'.

There is also the aspect of 'I shouldn't need to ask…' that comes with seniority and its implied higher level of experience. However, I have had several coaching sessions where the coach did a great job of helping me explore my issue, possible routes forward, and agreed a detailed plan (where, when, etc.) and even said something like 'I'll expect an email from you on Thursday at 1 pm to let me know how you've got on' – only to be allowed to get away with upholding my part of the bargain.

We all need to be accountable to someone for anything that we take seriously. This is not about being nagged; it is about being made to really commit to something, and then supported when we do not follow through, for whatever reason. However, nagging might be just what we need: I once hired someone to phone me at random intervals throughout a week of writing assignments!

Mentoring

The Mentoring phase stands for itself. Often I am coaching a leader of a team, and have some useful experience that I can draw on, even if it is not exactly in the same context.

Encouragement

The last phase is perhaps the most important. We all need someone to cheer for us, to urge us on, to encourage us to keep going in life, which can be full of 'aridity and disenchantment', as Max Ehrmann put it in 'Desiderata'.

Next steps

1. Do you need a coach or mentor? What are your objectives to work on together, are they more for mentoring or coaching? Who can you ask to find out what is available within your organisation, or outside of it?
2. Have you coaching and/or mentoring skills that you could use to build someone else's resilience? If you have the skills, make them available to others.

Afterword

The path ahead

'I love those who can smile in trouble, who can gather strength from distress, and grow brave by reflection. 'Tis the business of little minds to shrink, but they whose heart is firm, and whose conscience approves their conduct, will pursue their principles unto death.'

Leonardo da Vinci

As anyone reading this who has written their own book knows, a writer's emotions can swing rapidly from delight to despair. I thought it was just me, until I talked it through with my editor, Sue Richardson. One specific day taken from my journal encapsulates this.

I was struggling to climb and rework what is now Chapter 8 on drivers, and could not make progress. Seeking an example that might be closer to the world of policing, I opened John Sutherland's *Blue: A Memoir – Keeping the Peace, and Falling to Pieces* (2017) once again, and reread a large swathe of it. I was left saddened by the apparent hopelessness of so many situations in the London boroughs, the raw animal behaviour of some people and the desperation of others – all of which officers like John see every day for their entire careers.

Needing a change of scene, I climbed to my attic room and stuck my head out of the window, scaring pigeons from the tree outside off to chase friends and hopeful conquests. The traffic built and subsided in unnatural waves on the tarmac shore of the street below, as the breeze wafted the leaves about. The air was fresh and cleared my head a bit, exposing the deeper thoughts within.

Who am I kidding? How can I write of resilience to those who have had to deal with such situations? How dare I! Am I going to stir a hornets' nest of antagonistic backlash, that I have oversimplified or brushed aside the complexities of things that I have only experienced vicariously? Numb with pointlessness, I wondered: 'What now?' Deep breath. 'I have to finish this. Maybe even this little reflection will make its way into the book' – and indeed it has.

I hope that there are some useful ideas here. I hope that you can find even a small thing that you can try to use to build your own resilience, or get through yet another tricky situation. As I have written it, I too have been exploring some aspects of resilience in new ways.

I believe that everyone should be able to enjoy, not just endure, their work. That as leaders we owe it to ourselves to enable our people to thrive through what they do. However, all the topics we have explored together here may appear to be potentially expensive to implement.

When you consider unhelpful behaviours that we sometimes see at work – whether that is in terms of change, complaints, rumour and gossip, errors or just time loss – and you add up the small improvements that can be made every day then compare it to the salary bill for those involved, the investment of a few thousand pounds could save you potentially more than that per person.

It might look expensive in the short term, but it is a lot cheaper than the alternative cost of backfilling just one senior leader – and that is without factoring in the obvious costs of absence and long-term sickness.

As has been often repeated elsewhere: if you want a different result, take a different action.

Final reflection

1. What has particularly struck you as you have read this book?
2. Why is that significant to you?
3. What are you going to do now?

Resources

Workplace Resilience Instrument (WRI)

Mallak, L.A. (2018) Workplace Resilience Instrument (WRI).
Permission granted by copyright holder on 14 May, 2018.

	Not true at all	Rarely true	Sometimes true	Often true	True nearly all the time
I enjoy improvising solutions to problems.	1	2	3	4	5
I take delight in solving difficult problems.	1	2	3	4	5
I consider many feasible solutions when solving a problem.	1	2	3	4	5
Team goals guide my individual actions.	1	2	3	4	5
I show confidence in decisions affecting my team.	1	2	3	4	5
I discuss team member roles with my team members.	1	2	3	4	5
I understand my team's overall goals.	1	2	3	4	5
I approach new situations with confidence.	1	2	3	4	5
I try to make sense of the situation when it becomes chaotic.	1	2	3	4	5
I know what resources to access.	1	2	3	4	5
I openly share information with others.	1	2	3	4	5
I can perform the roles of my other team members.	1	2	3	4	5
I have access to the resources I need.	1	2	3	4	5
I have the knowledge needed to do my job.	1	2	3	4	5
I exercise creativity when under extreme pressure.	1	2	3	4	5
When a situation becomes chaotic, I am able to make sense of it.	1	2	3	4	5
When a situation becomes chaotic, I approach it as a challenge.	1	2	3	4	5
When a situation becomes chaotic, I get a renewed focus on the problem.	1	2	3	4	5
I take calculated risks when the situation calls for it.	1	2	3	4	5
When the situation becomes chaotic, I take time to reflect on next steps.	1	2	3	4	5

Scoring instructions

The Workplace Resilience Instrument (WRI) is scored across four factors:

1. Active problem-solving
2. Team efficacy
3. Confident sense-making
4. Bricolage.

Factor scores
Active problem-solving:

Sum the scores from items 1 to 3, and divide by 3: _____

Team efficacy:
Sum the scores from items 4 to 7, and divide by 4: _____

Confident sense-making:
Sum the scores from items 8 to 14, and divide by 7: _____

Bricolage:
Sum the scores from items 15 to 20, and divide by 6: _____

Although not defined theoretically, you may wish to compute an overall resilience score by either averaging the scores from each of the four factors, or by finding the average score across all 20 items: _____

Quick reference
While every section is relevant to building your resilience, the table below may help you identify which section(s) would be most useful to you from your scores in the WRI.

Low score in: Active problem-solving:

Chapter	
4	Purpose
5	Inner maps
6	Inner voice
7	Reframing

Chapter	
10	Mindset and motivation
11	Attitude and adversity
23	Feedback

Low score in: Team efficacy:

Chapter	
4	Purpose
5	Inner maps
6	Inner voice
8	What is driving you?
9	Temperament
12	Peak effectiveness times
13	Discipline, habits and practice
14	Planning
15	Distractions
16	Prioritisation
20	Self-compassion
21	Recuperation, rest and sleep
22	Connection
23	Feedback
24	Coaching and mentoring
25	Physical environment
26	Margin and the overload problem
27	Boundaries

Low score in: Confident sense-making:

Chapter	
7	Reframing
8	What is driving you?
9	Temperament
11	Attitude and adversity
14	Planning
15	Distractions
16	Prioritisation
18	Mindfulness
19	Reflection
26	Margin and the overload problem
27	Boundaries

Low score in: Bricolage:

Chapter	
10	Mindset and motivation
12	Peak effectiveness times
13	Discipline, habits and practice
18	Mindfulness
19	Reflection
22	Connection
24	Coaching and mentoring
25	Physical environment

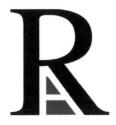 As a reader of this book, I would like to invite you to join the 'Resilience Alliance' – an informal alliance of individuals who are committed to improving their own, and others' resilience. As a member, you'll have access to all the additional materials mentioned throughout the book, and will receive a quarterly newsletter including updates and brief summaries of the latest research into resilience and stress applicable to individuals and teams.

Join me and many others by signing up at the-resilience-toolkit.com and get your copy of the Resilience Alliance manifesto 'The ReAll Manifesto'.

Introduction

Broderick, J. (2013) 'Trusting one's emotional guidance builds resilience'. In: V. Pulla, A. Shatté and S. Warren (eds.). *Perspectives on Coping and Resilience*. 1st ed. pp. 265. New Delhi: Authorspress.

Duckworth, A. (2016) *Grit: Why passion and resilience are the secrets to success*. UK: Penguin Random House.

Dweck, Dr C. (2012) *Mindset: How you can fulfil your potential*. Robinson, London.

Farmer, P. and Stevenson, D. (2017) 'Thriving at work: The Stevenson/Farmer review of mental health and employers'. p. 19. Available at: https://assets. publishing.service.gov.uk/government/uploads/system/uploads/attachment_data/file/658145/thriving-at-work-stevenson-farmer-review.pdf. Accessed June 2018.

Fletcher, D. and Sarkar, M. (2013) 'Psychological Resilience: A review and critique of definitions, concepts and theory'. *European Psychologist* 18(1), pp. 12–23. DOI: 10.1027/1016-9040/a000124.

Luthar, S., Cicchetti, D. and Becker, B. (2000) 'The construct of resilience: a critical evaluation and guidelines for future work'. *Child Development* 71(3), pp. 543–562.

Mallak, L. (2018) Workplace Resilience Instrument (WRI).

Mallak, L. and Yildiz, M. (2016) 'The development of a workplace resilience instrument'. *Work: A Journal of Prevention, Assessment and Rehabilitation* 54(2), pp. 241–253.

McCraty, R. and Atkinson, M. (2012) 'Resilience training program reduces physiological and psychological stress in police officers'. *Global Advances in Health and Medicine* 1(5), pp. 44–66. Available at: https://doi.org/10.7453/gahmj.2012.1.5.013.

'Myelin'. *Wikipedia.* Available at: https://en.wikipedia.org/wiki/Myelin. Accessed 25 October 2018.

Rutter, M. (2012) 'Resilience as a dynamic concept'. *Development and Psychopathology* 24, pp. 335–344. DOI: 10.1017/S0954579412000028.

Warner, R. and April, K. (2012) Building Personal Resilience at Work. *Effective Executive* 15(4), pp. 53–68.

Part 1: An integrated model

1. Background

Bandura, A. (1986) *Social Foundations of Thought and Action: A social cognitive theory*. Englewood Cliffs, NJ: Prentice-Hall.

Robertson, I., Cooper, C., Sarkar, M. and Curran, T. (2015) 'Resilience training in the workplace from 2003 to 2014: A systematic review'. *Journal of Occupational and Organizational Psychology* 88(3). Available at: doi.org/10.1111/joop.12120. Accessed 15 October 2018.

Weiten,W., Lloyd, M.A. and Dunn, D. (2008) *Psychology Applied to Modern Life: Adjustment in the 21st Century*. 9th ed. Wadsworth: Cengage Learning.

2. A resilience factor

Cooperrider D., Zandee D., Godwin L., Avital M. and Boland B. (eds.). (2013) *Organizational Generativity: The Appreciative Inquiry Summit and a Scholarship of Transformation (Advances in Appreciative Inquiry)*. Vol. 4, xi–xix. Emerald Group Publishing Limited.

Mallak, L. and Yildiz, M. (2016) 'The development of a workplace resilience instrument'. *Work: A Journal of Prevention, Assessment and Rehabilitation* 54(2), pp. 241–253.

Sun Tzu. (2009) *The Art of War*. Available at: http://classics.mit.edu//Tzu/artwar.html. Accessed 15 October 2018.

3. Compounding

Hieatt, D. (2014) 'Manifesto of a Doer'. Available at: http://davidhieatt.typepad.com/doonethingwell/2014/12/a-manifesto-of-a-doer.html. Accessed 15 October 2018

Part 2: Cognitive factors

4. Purpose

Campbell, J. (2009) 'Resilience in Personal and Organisational Life'. Available at: http://www.lifetimeswork.com/assets/documents/Insights/Insight%20 4%20Resilience%20Summary%20FINAL.pdf. Accessed 27 November 2018.

Covey, S. (2004) *The 7 Habits of Highly Effective People: Powerful lessons in personal change*. London: Simon & Schuster.

DoLectures. 'Purpose Matters'. Excerpt from 'The Stress Report'. Available at: https://medium.com/do-reports/purpose-matters-981937c8391. Accessed 24 October 2018.

Fixx, J. (1979) *The complete book of running*. London: Chatto & Windus.

O'Connor, J. and Seymour, J. (1995) *Introducing NLP: Psychological skills for understanding and influencing people*. p. 77. London: Thorsons.

Owen, N. (2001) *The Magic of Metaphor*. p. 14. Crown House Publishing Ltd.

Sinek, S. (2009) *Start with Why: How great leaders inspire everyone to take action*. London: Portfolio Penguin.

5. Inner maps

Charvet, S.R. (1997) *Words that Change Minds: Mastering the language of influence*. pp. 22. Kendall/Hunt Publishing.

Korzybski, A. (1995) *Science and Sanity: An introduction to non-aristotelian systems and general semantics*. 5th ed. Institute of General Semantics, Massachusetts.

Reivich, K. and Shatté, A. (2003) *The Resilience Factor: 7 keys to finding your inner strength and overcoming life's hurdles*. p. 66. Broadway books.

6. Inner voice

April, K. and Peters, K. (2012) 'Impact of Locus of Control Expectancy on Level of Well-Being'. *Review of European Studies* 4(2), pp. 124–137. DOI: 10.5539/res.v4n2p124.

Brown, B. (2015) *Rising Strong: How the ability to reset transforms the way we live, love, parent, and lead*. Spiegel & Grau.

Goleman, D. (1996) *Emotional Intelligence: Why it can matter more than IQ*. London: Bloomsbury.

Peters, S. (2013) *The Chimp Paradox: The acclaimed mind management programme to help you achieve success, confidence and happiness*. Ebury Publishing. Kindle Edition.

Pulla, V. and Shatté, A. (2013) 'Contours of coping and resilience'. *Perspectives on Coping and Resilience*. p. 18. Authorspress.

Rossouw, P. (2011) 'The Neuroscience of Depression'. Paper presentation at the Mediros Clinical Solutions, Sydney. *Perspectives on Coping and Resilience*. p. 101.

7. Reframing

Collins, J. (2001) *Good to Great: Why some companies make the leap… and others don't*. p. 85. New York: HarperCollins.

Epictetus. (1888) *The Enchiridion, or Handbook: With a selection from the discourses of Epictetus*. p. 271. Auckland: The Floating Press.

Stoeber, J. and Jansen, D. (2011) 'Perfectionism and Coping With Daily Failures: Positive reframing helps achieve satisfaction at the end of the day'. *Anxiety, Stress and Coping* 24(5), pp. 477–497. DOI: 10.1080/10615806.2011.562977.

8. What is driving you?

Hay, J. (2012) *Transactional Analysis for Trainers*. pp. 95. UK: Sherwood Publishing.

Kahler, T. (1978) *Transactional analysis revisited*. Little Rock: Human Development Publications.

Tice, D.M. and Baumeister, R.F. (1997) 'Longitudinal Study of Procrastination, Performance, Stress, and Health: The costs and benefits of dawdling'. *Psychological Science* 8(6), pp. 454–458. Available at: https://doi.org/10.1111/j.1467-9280.1997.tb00460.x.

9. Temperament

Keirsey, D. (1998) *Please Understand Me II: Temperament, character, intelligence*. Del Mar, USA: Prometheus Nemesis Book Company.

10. Mindset and motivation

Dweck, Dr C. (2012) *Mindset: The new psychology of success*. London: Robinson.

'Frederick Winslow Taylor'. *Wikipedia*. Available at: https://en.wikipedia.org/wiki/Frederick_Winslow_Taylor. Accessed 22 October 2018.

Packard, D. (1995) *The HP Way: How Bill Hewlett and I built our company*. London: Harper Business.

Pink, D. (2010) *Drive: The surprising truth about what motivates us*. London: Canongate Books.

11. Attitude and adversity

Conner, D.R. (1992) *Managing at the Speed of Change: How resilient managers succeed and prosper where others fail*. Toronto: Random House.

Epictetus. (1877) *The Discourses of Epictetus: With the Encheiridion and fragments*. p. 5. Chesterfield soc.

Frankl, V. (2004) *Man's search for meaning: The classic tribute to hope from the Holocaust*. London: Rider.

Poynton, R. (2008) *Everything's an Offer: How to do more with less*. Portland, Oregon: On Your Feet.

Seligman, M.E.P. (2011) *Flourish*. Nicholas Brealey Publishing.

Warren, S. (2013) 'Revisiting emotional regulation: Evidence from practice'. In: V. Pulla, A. Shatté and S. Warren (eds.). *Perspectives on Coping and Resilience*. 1st ed. p. 388. New Delhi: Authorspress.

Wheatley, A.M. (2013) 'Building resilience in the next generation and the power of higher self-efficacy'. In: V. Pulla, A. Shatté and S. Warren (eds.). *Perspectives on Coping and Resilience.* 1st ed. pp. 365–366. New Delhi: Authorspress.

Wheatley, A.M. (2011) 'The impact of self-efficacy and challenge/threat evaluations on academic procrastination'. Thesis (unpublished). Postgraduate Diploma of Psychological studies, University of Western Sydney, New South Wales, Australia. As referenced in A.M. Wheatley. (2013) 'Building resilience in the next generation and the power of higher self-efficacy'. In: V. Pulla, A. Shatté and S. Warren (eds.). *Perspectives on Coping and Resilience.* 1st ed. pp. 365–366. New Delhi: Authorspress.

Williams, M.T. (2015) *Do Breathe: Calm your mind. Find focus. Get stuff done.* The Do Book Company Ltd.

Part 3: Behavioural factors

12. Peak effectiveness times

Goldsmith, M. and Reiter, M. (2016) *Triggers: Sparking positive change and making it last.* London: Profile Books Ltd.

Newport, C. (2016) *Deep Work: Rules for focused success in a distracted world.* London: Piatkus.

Penn, W. (1693) 'Some fruits of solitude'. *A Collection of the Works of William Penn: To which is prefixed a journal of his life, with many original letters and papers not before published.* Assigns of J. Sowle.

Pink, D.H. (2018) *When: The scientific secrets of perfect timing.* pp. 26, 53, 96. Edinburgh: Canongate Books Ltd.

13. Discipline, habits and practice

Brannaman, B. (2003) *Faraway Horses: The adventures and wisdom of one of America's most renowned horsemen.* Lyons Press.

Duhigg, C. (2012) *The Power of Habit: Why we do what we do in life and business.* Pretoria Books.

Levitin, D.J. (2006) *This is Your Brain On Music: The science of a human obsession.* pp. 197. New York: Dutton.

The Bible. 1 Corinthians 9:25–27. English Standard Version (ESV).

14. Planning

Chesney, C. (2012) *The 4 Disciplines of Execution: Achieving your wildly important goals.* London: Simon & Schuster.

Gollwitzer, A., Oettingen, G., Kirby, T.A., Duckworth, A.L. and Mayer, D. (2011) 'Mental contrasting facilitates academic performance in school children'. *Motivation and Emotion* 35, pp. 403–412.

Tracy, B. (2003) *Eat That Frog! Twenty-one great ways to stop procrastinating and get more done in less time.* p. 17. San Francisco: Berrett-Koehler Publishers Inc.

15. Distractions

Alter, A. (2017) *Irresistible: The rise of addictive technology and the business of keeping us hooked.* New York: Penguin press.

Astle, D.E., Jackson, G.M. and Swainson, R. (2006) 'Dissociating neural indices of dynamic cognitive control in advance task-set preparation: an ERP study of task switching'. *Brain Res.* 1125(1) pp. 94–103.

Holesh, K. (2014) *Moment.* Mobile application. https://inthemoment.io. Accessed 15 October 2018. Usage data kindly provided personally on 10 December 2018.

KPCB. (2018) 'Internet Trends Report 2018'. Available at: http://www.kpcb.com/internet-trends. Accessed 15 October 2018.

Leroy, S. (2009) 'Why Is It So Hard to Do My Work? The Challenge of Attention Residue When Switching Between Work Tasks.' Organizational Behavior and Human Decision Processes 109(2) pp. 168–181.

Newport, C. (2016) *Deep Work: Rules for focused success in a distracted world.* London: Piatkus.

Ophir, E., Nass, C. and Wagner, A.D. (2009) 'Cognitive control in media multitaskers'. Available at: https://www.pnas.org/content/106/37/15583. Accessed 15 October 2018.

Perlow, L.A. and Porter, J.L. (2009) 'Making Time Off Predictable – and Required'. *Harvard Business Review.* October. Available at: https://hbr.org/2009/10/making-time-off-predictable-and-required. Accessed 15 October 2018.

Rock, D. (2009) *Your Brain at Work: Strategies for overcoming distraction, regaining focus, and working smarter all day long.* HarperCollins.

Rogers, R.D. and Monsell, S. (1995) 'The costs of a predictable switch between simple cognitive tasks'. *Journal of Experimental Psychology General* 124(2) pp. 207–231.

16. Prioritisation

Federation of American Scientists. (n.a.) 'Appendix D: Target analysis process'. Available at: https://fas.org/irp/doddir/army/fm34-36/appd.htm. Accessed 25 October 2018.

'MoSCoW method'. *Wikipedia*. Available at: https://en.wikipedia.org/wiki/MoSCoW_method. Accessed 4 December 2018.

Mueller, P.A. and Oppenheimer, D.M. (2014) 'The Pen Is Mightier Than the Keyboard: Advantages of longhand over laptop note taking'. *Psychological Science* 25(6), pp. 1159–1168. Available at: https://doi.org/10.1177/0956797614524581. Accessed 15 October 2018.

Rock, D. (2009) *Your Brain at Work: Strategies for overcoming distraction, regaining focus, and working smarter all day long.* HarperCollins.

17. Exercise

Fixx, J. (1979) *The complete book of running.* pp. xiv. London: Chatto & Windus.

Rebar, A.L., Stanton, R., Geard, D., Short, C., Duncan, M.J. and Vandelanotte, C. (2015) 'A meta-meta-analysis of the effect of physical activity on depression and anxiety in non-clinical adult populations'. *Health Psychology Review* 9(3), 366e378. Available at: https://doi.org/10.1080/17437199.2015.1022901. Accessed 15 October 2018.

18. Mindfulness

Berman, M.G., Jonides, J. and Kaplan, S. (2008) 'The cognitive benefits of interacting with nature'. *Psychological Science* 19(12), pp. 1207–1212. Available at: https://doi.org/10.1111/j.1467-9280.2008.02225.x. Accessed 15 October 2018.

Davis, D.M. and Hayes, J.A. (2012) 'What are the benefits of mindfulness: A wealth of new research has explored this age-old practice. Here's a look at its benefits for both clients and psychologists'. *American Psychological Association*. Available at https://www.apa.org/monitor/2012/07-08/ce-corner.aspx. Accessed 15 October 2018.

Hunt, C. (2016) *What Trauma Taught Me about Resilience*. TEDx Talk, Charlotte. Available at: youtube.com/watch?v=3qELiw_1Ddg. Accessed 15 October 2018.

19. Reflection

Berends, P.B. (1990) *Coming to Life: Travelling the spiritual path in everyday life.* San Francisco: HarperCollins.

Kelly, J. (2012) 'Resilience building using art therapy with adolescents in Australia'. In: V. Pulla, A. Shatté and S. Warren (eds.). *Perspectives on Coping and Resilience.* 1st ed. pp. 159–166. New Delhi: Authorspress.

Pink, D.H. (2018) *When: The scientific secrets of perfect timing.* Edinburgh: Canongate Books Ltd.

Seligman, M.E.P. (2011) *Flourish*. Nicholas Brealey Publishing.

20. Self-compassion

Knight, S. (2017) *You Do You: How to be who you are and use what you've got to get what you want*. Quercus.

Neff, K.D., Long, P., Knox, M.C., Davidson, O., Kuchar, A., Costigan, A. and Williamson, Z. (2018) 'The Forest and the Trees: Examining the factor structure of the self-compassion scale and the association of its positive and negative components with psychological functioning'. *Self and Identity*. Available at: https://doi.org/10.1080/15298868.2018.1436587. Accessed 15 October 2018.

The Bible. Philippians 4:12 and Galatians 5:22–23. New International Version (NIV).

Winch, G. (2014) *Why We All Need to Practice Emotional First Aid*. TEDx Talk, Linnaeus University. Available at: ted.com/talks/guy_winch_the_case_for_emotional_hygiene?language=en. Accessed 15 October 2018.

21. Recuperation, rest and sleep

Edwards, B. (1992) *Drawing on the Right Side of the Brain: A course in enhancing creativity and artistic confidence*. London: HarperCollins.

'Effect of psychoactive drugs on animals'. *Wikipedia*. Available at: https://en.wikipedia.org/wiki/Effect_of_psychoactive_drugs_on_animals. Accessed 4 December 2018.

Ehrmann, M. (1952) 'Desiderata'. Available at: http://mwkworks.com/desiderata.html. Accessed 10 December 2018.

Kelly, J. (2012) 'Resilience building using art therapy with adolescents in Australia'. In: V. Pulla, A. Shatté and S. Warren (eds.). *Perspectives on Coping and Resilience*. 1st ed. p. 159. New Delhi: Authorspress.

Mudaly, N., Graham, A. and Lewis, N. (2014) '"It takes me a little longer to get angry now": Homeless children traumatised by family violence reflect on an animal therapy group'. *Children Australia*.

Pennebaker, J.W., Kiecolt-Glaser, J.K. and Glaser, R. (1988) 'Disclosure of traumas and immune function: Health implications for psychotherapy'. *Journal of Consulting and Clinical Psychology* 56, pp. 239–245.

PFOA. (2017) 'Trauma Risk Management (TRiM)'. Available at: https://www.pfoa.co.uk/support/trauma-risk-management-trim. Accessed 24 October 2018.

Roberts, R. and Thomas, M. The Zentangle® Method. Available at: zentangle. com.

'Seneca the Younger'. *WikiQuote*. 'On tranquillity of mind'. Available at: https:// en.wikiquote.org/wiki/Seneca_the_Younger. Accessed 24 October 2018.

Spurgeon, C. (1856) 'Lecture XI'. *Lectures to My Students: Volume 1*. pp. 178–179. Available at: https://www.mat.univie.ac.at/~neum/sciandf/spurgeon/spurgeon1.pdf. Accessed 24 October 2018.

Walker, M. (2018) *Why We Sleep*. London: Penguin.

Part 4: Relational factors

22. Margin and the overload problem

Swenson, R.A. (2004) *Margin: Restoring emotional, physical, financial, and time reserves to overloaded lives*. NavPress.

23. Boundaries

Cloud, H. and Townsend, J. (1992) *Boundaries: When to say yes, how to say no*. Michigan: Zondervan.

Feynman, R. (1988) 'Nobel Physicist R. P. Feynman of Caltech Dies'. *Los Angeles Times*. Available at: http://articles.latimes.com/1988-02-16/news/mn-42968_1_nobel-prize/2. Accessed 24 October 2018.

24. Physical environment

Goldsmith, M. and Reiter, M. (2016) *Triggers: Sparking positive change and making it last*. London: Profile Books Ltd.

25. Connection

Betancourt, I., et al. (2012) Quoted in White, A. and Pulla V. 'Strengthening the capacity for resilience in children'. In: V. Pulla, A. Shatté and S. Warren (eds.). *Perspectives on Coping and Resilience*. 1st ed. p. 138. New Delhi: Authorspress.

26. Feedback

Feynman, R. (1992) *"Surely You're Joking, Mr. Feynman!": Adventures of a curious character*. Vintage Books.

Kaye, B. and Jordan-Evans, S. (2005) *Love 'Em or Lose 'Em: Getting good people to stay*. Williston: Berrett-Koehler Publishers, Inc.

Marquet, D.L. (2012) *Turn the Ship Around! A true story of turning followers into leaders*. pp. 135–141. New York: Penguin.

27. Coaching and mentoring

McNeely, M. and Ehrenreich, M. (n.a.) 'How to adopt a coaching mentality and practice'. *Harvard Extension School: Professional Development*. Available at: https://www.extension.harvard.edu/professional-development/blog/how-adopt-coaching-mentality-and-practice. Accessed 24 October 2018.

Afterword

Sutherland, J. (2017) *Blue: A memoir – keeping the peace, and falling to pieces*. London: Weidenfeld & Nicolson.

In 2010, a few months after the death of my father, I took a redundancy package from Hewlett-Packard, bringing to an end an IT career spanning over two decades.

Starting as a graduate at British Aerospace, I was initially captivated by writing software, despite the personal computer being virtually unknown in the workplace at the time. We had one machine between 100 of us, and shared phones too!

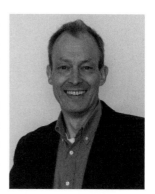

Following several moves, I ended up at HP, managing a team of 18 staff spread across three continents, and owning a portfolio of 24/7 applications with tens of thousands of users around the globe. I transitioned from that to IT consulting activities, working with companies on-site and off-site in the UK and abroad.

I now realise that all of these jobs had people at their core. After leaving IT I discovered that I was not a 'geek', just someone happy around technical things. If I did it all again, I'd probably choose a degree in psychology – technology of a different kind.

In 2017, after nearly eight years of running my own business facilitating and delivery workshops and coaching, I was invited to speak at the UK national conference of the Police Superintendents' Association. I was given an hour to 'provide something useful on resilience that delegates can take away and apply in their day job'.

Since then, I've travelled all over the UK and Ireland delivering workshops and keynote speeches to more than 600 police officers. My primary focus is now on working with people in the emergency services, enabling them to build more resilient lives for themselves and those they work with – in the hope that this will enable them to have more resilient families, neighbourhoods and communities.

Acknowledgements

I wish to thank:

Chief Superintendent Ian Wylie of Avon & Somerset Police for the idea to write this book, for his encouragement and enthusiasm, as well as writing the foreword. Also to Dr Larry Mallak for his permission to use his Workplace Resilience Instrument, and his painstaking review comments.

All those who provided comments on the drafts, including several police officers. You know who you are! And to the many researchers and authors whose work has inspired me and contributed to this book, especially Jenny Campbell, Dan Pink, John Sutherland and Kevin Holesh – who kindly provided up-to-the-minute data on phone usage.

Sonja Jefferson, Sharon Tanton and all at pub school and pub club. Sue Richardson (and her team at SRA Books) for her patient reviewing of my endless scribblings and shaping it into what you have before you. Mike Clarke for his great website copy and persistent questioning – 'And then what happens?' Christian Tait for turning around the graphics at short notice and in record time! My patient and loving family, Sue, Emily and Osian – sorry for the many times I skipped my washing-up duties to 'just go and write a bit more'.

And finally, Jesus Christ, the person who provides the foundation for my personal resilience, and helps me to live freely and lightly.